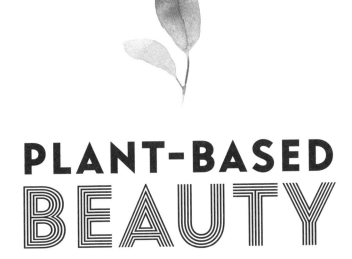

PLANT-BASED
BEAUTY

ASTER*

JESS ARNAUDIN

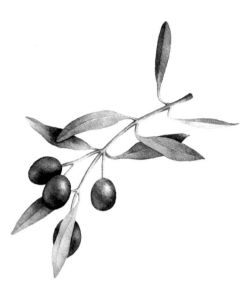

PLANT-BASED
BEAUTY

THE ESSENTIAL GUIDE TO DETOXING
YOUR BEAUTY ROUTINE

aster

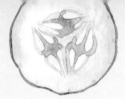

DEDICATION

For my daughters Anna and Julia

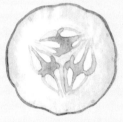

ASTER*

First published in Great Britain in 2018 by Aster,
an imprint of Octopus Publishing Group Ltd
Carmelite House
50 Victoria Embankment
London EC4Y 0DZ
www.octopusbooks.co.uk
www.octopusbooksusa.com

An Hachette UK Company
www.hachette.co.uk

This edition published in 2023

Text copyright © Jess Arnaudin 2019
Design and layout copyright © Octopus Publishing
Group Ltd 2019

Distributed in the US by
Hachette Book Group
1290 Avenue of the Americas
4th and 5th Floors
New York, NY 10104

Distributed in Canada by
Canadian Manda Group
664 Annette St.
Toronto, Ontario, Canada M6S 2C8

ISBN 978 1 78325 593 1

Printed and bound in China

10 9 8 7 6 5 4 3 2 1

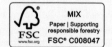

MIX
Paper | Supporting
responsible forestry
FSC® C008047

FSC
www.fsc.org

Consultant Publisher: Kate Adams
Senior Editor: Sophie Elletson
Designer: Geoff Fennell
Production Manager: Lisa Pinnell

CONTENTS

FOREWORD

Plant-Based Beauty is the perfect guidebook for anyone who feels called to learn more about what plant-based beauty means, why it's important, and how to incorporate plant-based beauty rituals into your everyday life. Jess Arnaudin walks you through her philosophy that plants have the powerful ability to heal your skin, based on her belief that 'nature is the master chemist'. When it comes to your food and your beauty products, I couldn't agree more. Through my personal journey and my work as a clean beauty makeup artist and founder of the Sacred Beauty Movement, I've seen firsthand how choosing a plant-based lifestyle benefits your skin's radiance and your overall vitality.

What's also important about this book is that it comes at a time when many people are becoming more conscious about what we eat, drink and think. This guide offers alternatives to fast food and fast beauty consumption by cultivating beauty through mindfulness. As Jess says so well in the introduction, 'The plant-based beauty mindset seeks to bring health and

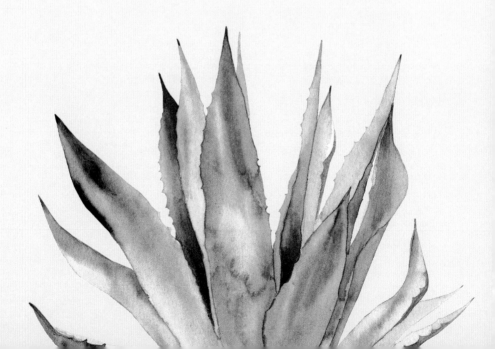

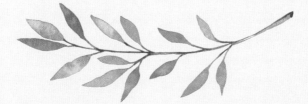

harmony to every function of your body. Emotional health; gentle exercise; a healing antioxidant-rich diet; a properly functioning digestive system; and a passion-driven mindful lifestyle; all combine to equal healthy, beautiful skin.' She understands the deep connection between our inner and outer beauty and helps us navigate the relationship with ease.

Jess is a passionate skin therapist, rooted in her deep love of nature, beauty and service. She truly wants to empower her clients and people worldwide with a holistic, plant-based approach to beauty. Her work draws on everything from ancient beauty secrets to cutting-edge spa treatments. From her skincare services, to this book you are holding in your hands, she aims to educate and inspire you with the tools to love the skin you're in. This book is packed with fresh ideas, practical knowledge and delicious, simple, beauty food recipes. I'm grateful to have *Plant-Based Beauty* in my library and I know you will be too. Heed the wisdom of Mother Nature and trust her process!

Wishing you a wonderful journey of self-discovery and abundant, natural, beauty,

Rebecca Casciano

Makeup Artist, Natural Beauty Expert and Founder of The Sacred Beauty Movement
The Sacred Beauty Movement was created to help women discover the connection between inner and outer beauty, love themselves more and uplift one another along the way. Together, we are creating a new, empowered beauty culture for generations to come. Learn more at *www.rebeccacasciano.com*.

INTRODUCTION

A PERSONAL JOURNEY OF INSPIRATION

West of the Hudson River and nestled among the majestic Catskill Mountains of New York is a small town called Kingston. Within this adorable little town is an organic farm that changed the course of my life forever.

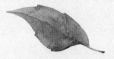

I was four years into my career as a skincare therapist in New York City when I began to feel a tug toward a simpler, more beauty-filled life. My husband and I lived in a tiny studio apartment in the East Village of Manhattan and, despite a few failed attempts at growing our own herbs on the fire escape, or 'harvesting' our own wheatgrass for smoothies from a plastic tray that took up the entire worktop, we knew very little about 'green living' at first. But in New York you can find out about just about anything that interests you – that's exactly what I love most about the city.

We gradually discovered small enclaves of revolutionaries who cared about the environment, kept bees on rooftops, and understood the rhythms of the growing seasons – even in the shadows of high-rise, glimmering buildings. On the weekends, we'd travel to Governor's Island to help tend to chickens (and one very stubborn goat) and we listened to talks about vermiculture (composting with worms) and the importance of seed saving. I joined a group in Brooklyn committed to swapping goods and attended one of their gatherings. It was the most wonderful experience! I arrived with 26 jars of apple jam made in my own tiny kitchen and returned home with homemade ginger sweets, fermented kohlrabi, spicy mustard and a cornucopia of other delights that were altogether so exotic and exciting to me.

This life felt like such a stark contrast to the 9–5 experience of working at a popular spa on Fifth Avenue. While I was grateful for the job, it felt vapid. Back then, I was only dealing with the surface – the skin's epidermis to be exact. Clients came in with high hopes for turning back the clock in an hour. We peeled, scrubbed, scraped, waxed, pricked, squeezed and injected. There was no mind–body connection. There was no element of respect for the innate beauty found in imperfection. We sold the ideal. We sold jars filled with promises and pseudo-miracles.

Distinctly, I remember one evening on the way home from work, I boarded the train and broke down into tears. I knew I had to change my path. I knew there had to be more to the beauty industry than frothy, superficial quick fixes. It felt dishonest and unhealthy and I was ready for what was wholesome and true.

One month later, my husband drove me three hours north of the city in a rental car, with our chestnut-brown beagle laid over my lap in the passenger seat. We pulled into the dirt driveway that led to the organic farm that I'd be living on for the next 30 days through a work-exchange programme. My husband was committed in the city, but he promised to visit on the weekends and supported my agrarian dream. Quickly, that dream became a reality as I began to learn first-hand the work involved in operating a farm. But the authenticity and beauty of the land far outweighed the exhausting back-breaking labour. For the first time, I sincerely understood what it meant to feel connected to the earth. The host family I lived with was an inspiration and study in what it means to be self-sustaining. They ate bright yellow eggs from their own chickens, baked fresh bread daily, stored root vegetables in the cellar and chopped wood for a stove that heated the entire house. The warmth greeted you like a hug.

Two weeks into living this way, I noticed a change in my own skin. It glowed with health. There were no retinoids or chemical peels on the farm, and yet my chronic skin inflammation and jawline breakouts were diminishing. There was a cold-pressed red raspberry seed oil that I applied to

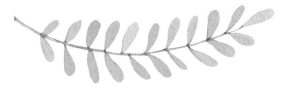

my skin each night by candlelight and raw honey from the local bees that I used every few days as a mask on my wind-chapped skin. It may sound insane, but I remember harvesting rocket in the rain one cold morning and I could literally feel the vibration of pure energy radiating from the earth. I remember turning my face skyward and yelling, 'I am a warrior princess!' Thank goodness I was alone at the time, otherwise my hosts might have thought I'd lost my marbles. But something there awakened me, and opened my eyes to the beauty, potency and wisdom of plants.

There was no doubt that I would take this reverence for plants (and the hands that grow them) back home with me. When I returned home to NYC, I accepted a job at an adorable organic spa in the West Village. From then on, I spent my days ravenously learning about plants that nourish, exfoliate, protect and heal the skin.

Nearly a decade into this journey as a skin therapist, I now understand that one of the biggest differences in conventional skincare versus plant-based beauty comes down to a subtle shift in philosophy. Many big-name beauty brands keep the revenue streaming in by planting seeds of doubt and by indirectly encouraging the universal fear that you need to be fixed in some way, shape or form; that your skin is not capable of health without the newest product launch. How many times have we heard or read this in some iteration: 'buy THIS and your skin will be prettier' or 'your hair will be bouncier'. In some ways, mainstream beauty dogma tells us that, in order to be loved, we must manage our misbehaving skin with whatever magic potion they're selling. As women, especially, we hold ourselves up to an impossible standard, heightened and more sharply defined by the media to which we are exposed.

In addition to this – believe me – there is a never-ending cascade of buying more to feel more worthy. As an ex-product junkie myself, my surfaces were cluttered and my bathroom drawers overflowed with all kinds

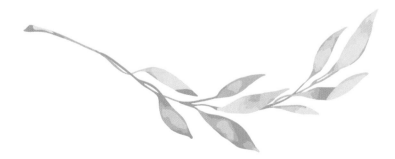

of make-up and skincare. Yet, even though this excess surrounded me, it never felt like I had enough. That was until I began to truly embrace the fundamentals of skin health (spoiler alert: it's not found at the bottom of an expensive face cream) and how to care for my skin with less. Fewer ingredients, fewer products, less negative self-talk.

The plant-based beauty mindset seeks to bring health and harmony to *every* function of your body. Emotional health; gentle exercise; a healing antioxidant-rich diet; a properly functioning digestive system; and a passion-driven mindful lifestyle; all combine to equal healthy, beautiful skin. This isn't a checklist to pressure you into perfectionism, but rather an invitation to view your body through a holistic lens, and cultivating more kindness toward yourself and your skin as a result.

This book is my gratitude journal to the plants that forever changed the way I care for my skin and my clients' skin. In many ways, we've forgotten the wisdom of our ancestors. We've stared at our smart devices and turned up the TV so as not to hear the gentle stirrings of the natural world. From the blue glow of our screens, we are bombarded by wave-upon-wave of marketing claims promising pore-less, 'blemish'-free skin overnight. However, through gentle beauty routines, practical suggestions and powerfully pure products, I'm hopeful that you will walk away from this book viewing your skin as a living organ that sometimes requires healing, not hiding. May these self-care tips, beauty food recipes, and plant-based skincare concoctions be a compassionate counter-cultural salve for your skin and soul.

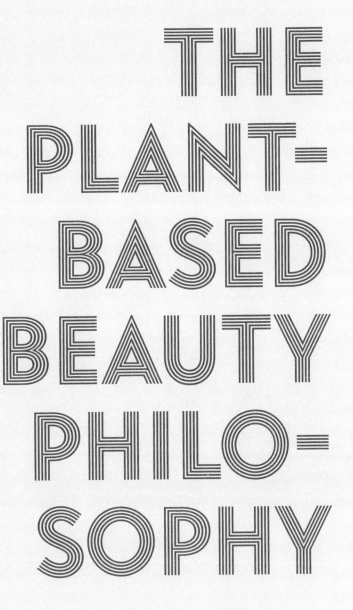

THE PLANT-BASED BEAUTY PHILOSOPHY

NATURE IS THE MASTER CHEMIST

Nature knows best. Plant-based beauty recipes, made with roots, fruits, flowers, herbs and nut and seed oils, contain powerful phytochemicals. *Wait... what? You're telling me there are chemicals in my organic plant-based products?* Of course there are! Marketing efforts would have you believe 'chemicals' are the enemy, when, of course, all matter is made up of chemicals. Everything we breathe, see, touch, eat, and apply to our skin is chemical-based. It's our job to make sure these are friendly, non-carcinogenic compounds that nourish the skin, rather than cause damage. And that's where time-tested, hard-working plants come in. Believe this: unrefined, organic, plant-powered skincare will transform your skin. When you experience this type of skin healing, you'll never want to go back to processed ingredients that are made synthetically in the lab and devoid of colour.

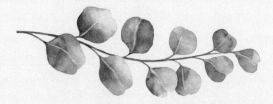

Take vibrant sea buckthorn oil, for example. Just one bright-orange drop contains carotenoids, such as beta-carotene and lycopene, which protect against sun damage. It also contains vitamins A, C and E, and a generous mix of B vitamins and essential fatty acids, which balance dry skin, soothe burns and help to clear acne-prone skin. This is the intricate, powerful science of Nature. While man-made synthetic skincare is not all inherently bad for your skin or health, I do believe Nature to be the master chemist. Often, skincare companies will add synthetic fragrances, parabens, fillers, alcohols and 'plant-identical' ingredients because it is more cost-effective and the skincare remains more shelf stable. The bottom line is monetary profit, not necessarily what benefits you or your skin the most.

We live in a culture that celebrates hyper-efficiency. We are always trying to find more ways to multi-task and get the same result in less time. This is all well and good in certain applications; however, when it comes to our skincare we tend to place the same expectation on our products and getting instant overnight results. Couple this with the fact that products are being manufactured faster and more cheaply to keep up with the demand of the beauty industry – essentially, what we are left with is a high-consumption 'fast food' skincare landscape.

Think of your raw plant-based skincare as you would your food. We all know that filling our plates with fresh organic produce is amazing for our health – the cells of our bodies basically do a happy dance with each vibrant bite! Then, imagine canned vegetables that have been collecting dust on a shelf at your grocery store. Or, taking it even further, imagine eating non-food – those processed 'food-like' ingredients in packaged junk foods. You might gulp down some vitamins on top and call it a well-balanced meal? No way! It's clear that freshly picked, nutrient-dense, locally sourced plant foods are much more nourishing and beneficial. The same concept applies to your skincare. Plants are highly intelligent – trust them.

PLANT-BASED BEAUTY MYTHS

1 **Plant-based beauty is only for organic purists.
It's too restrictive and I won't be able to find clean
product swaps that compare to the ones I already use.**

False! Now more than ever, plant-based beauty is accessible to all and can easily be incorporated into your busy everyday routine. The natural beauty market is growing rapidly and independent brands have created incredibly luxurious, high-performing products that rival mainstream skincare and cosmetics. It's easier than ever to go green and clean!

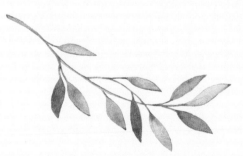

Sure, plant-based products may smell nice, but they don't deliver results.

False! Let's set the record straight once and for all. Many of the ingredients found in plant-based beauty products are similar to those in conventional formulations – only better! Plants naturally contain effective active ingredients that benefit your skin, such as alpha hydroxy acids (AHAs), fruit enzymes, vitamins A, C and E, polyphenols, hyaluronic acid, flavonoids, ferulic acid and carotenoids. Whole plant skincare is even *more* potent because it was perfected by nature. Much of what makes up traditional skincare is fillers, preservatives, scents, emulsifiers and additives that impact the texture, consistency and shelf life of the end product. These added extras provide no therapeutic value to the formula. However, in plant-based beauty, the products are much more concentrated and every last ingredient packs a powerful, purposeful punch.

I'd like to use more natural products, but plant-based beauty is always so expensive.

It's true that many independent plant-based beauty brands have skewed toward the luxury sector. This is due partially to the expenses of sourcing, harvesting and producing truly pure, plant-based products. But the good news is that, often, plant-based products end up being better value in the long run. Since the products are highly concentrated without chemical fillers, you'll end up needing to use much less.

If you think about the CPU – or *cost per use* – of plant-based beauty products, you'll find that the benefits over time are well worth the initial outlay. Let's reframe our buying habits and move from impulsive click-and-buy skincare purchases to well-researched, as they say in fashion, 'investment pieces' that will benefit your skin and health in the long term.

Within this book is a bevy of do-it-yourself recipes – some of which can be whipped up using as little as two ingredients from your kitchen! Other DIY recipes found here will require investing in a few sustainably sourced, whole plant raw materials. Either way, making your own products at home is almost always a cost-effective strategy.

INSIDE
OUT
BEAUTY

'BEAUTY
IS NOT IN
THE FACE;
BEAUTY
IS A LIGHT
IN THE
HEART.'

- KAHLIL GIBRAN

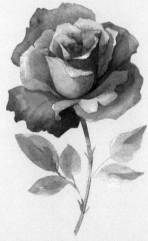

As a holistic skincare therapist, it's my job to consider the whole person. I'm not simply treating the symptoms of the skin with harsh peels, aggressive scrubs or lasers, but rather drawing from the ancient science of healing plants and acknowledging the deeper mind–body connection manifested through our skin. There is a time and a place for all therapies and I do not wish to villainize traditional esthetic practices; however, rarely are the root causes of skin symptoms explored before moving on with invasive resurfacing or dermabrasion procedures involving lasers or chemical peels.

If you've never experienced a facial with a holistic, plant-based skincare therapist, I encourage you to seek one out and book an appointment. A skilled therapist will be able to assess and coach you on the health of your skin, make lifestyle suggestions, and also treat you to an incredible facial massage. In holistic practices our hands are our main tools, along with non-invasive methods such as Gua sha stones, kansa wands, reflexology rollers, herbal poultices and facial cupping techniques. My ultimate goal is to create a safe, non-judgmental environment in the treatment room – a reprieve from the stresses of daily life, where clients can be vulnerable enough to ask questions and leave feeling empowered and inspired to continue caring for themselves at home through simple, meaningful self-care rituals. It's less about leading clients to buy a miracle cream, and more about lovingly encouraging an all-encompassing lifestyle, understanding that all parts are interconnected.

A MINDFUL EXERCISE

Let's explore this inside—out connection:

Even though your skin may be imbalanced, it isn't broken. Inherently, it doesn't need to be 'fixed' by the traditional definition. For just a moment, put aside the inner critic and remember that your skin, this amazing organ, keeps your body safe and balanced on its own (without any help). Skin regulates body temperature, provides a protective barrier, keeps vital organs hydrated, produces essential vitamin D, senses danger and delight via sensory receptors, secretes and excretes to keep the body healthy, and naturally produces melanin to protect you from scorching immediately in the sun. Think about it: if you accidentally cut your finger in the kitchen, your body will naturally synthesize new tissue and eventually mend on its own. Applying topical treatments will play a supportive role in fast-tracking your body's natural healing process, but they alone are not what restores your skin.

I earnestly believe that, if we begin our journey with understanding and immense gratitude for the physiological functions of our skin, we will be better able to discern what our skin needs and how to help it function with more health and vibrancy.

EXERCISE

Close your eyes and take a few deep inhalations. Become still and sit with your body (and your skin), being aware of exactly how it is in this moment. Surrender any ideas or standards of how you think your skin should look. Can you stir a feeling of gratitude and inner-compassion for your beautiful body, just as it is, *exactly in this moment*?

EAT TO NOURISH

GLOW FOODS FOR RADIANT SKIN

The skin is your body's largest organ and it certainly reflects your inner health. What you eat plays a vital role in skin health.

Your body craves organic, anti-inflammatory nutrients so that the skin can function optimally and glow from the inside out. I like to call these 'beauty foods' or 'glow foods' and I have provided a list of my favourites over the following pages. These foods work to slow down oxidation (hence the name 'antioxidants'), boost your immune system, restore the strength of your skin and promote healing. My list is certainly not an exhaustive one; rather it is a starter guide to the many beneficial foods that will nourish you from within.

My hope is that, once you adopt the plant-based beauty lifestyle, you'll have a better understanding of how your mind, body and spirit are all interconnected. With this understanding deep in your bones, you'll be empowered to choose foods that support you in living your best, most energetic and beautiful life. Here are my top beauty food suggestions to keep skin gorgeous and glowing.

CHOOSING FOODS MINDFULLY

When I worked on the farm, it opened my eyes to how vitally important it is to support local farmers who practise organic or biodynamic farming methods. Believe this: not all glow foods are created equally. Find a local farmers' or community producers' market. You'll get the highest amounts of antioxidants and micronutrients from in-season food grown on local farms that follow crop rotation, composting and organic pest management, and that harvest only when the crop is ripe (rather than allowing produce to 'ripen' in transit or – worse – via chemical ripening using calcium carbide).

VEGETABLES

There's no need to make a case for vegetables. Whether you're obsessed with all things veggie, or you have negative childhood memories of 'not leaving the table until you've finished your Brussels sprouts', most of us know that vegetables benefit our general health. But did you know that some vegetables are higher in skin-loving antioxidants and more beneficial than others?

SWEET POTATOES AND CARROTS

These two orange beauties both contain beta-carotene. When you ingest beta-carotene, your body converts it to vitamin A – it's Nature's retinol! You may have seen retinol in many mainstream skincare products, but eating this powerful antioxidant in its organic form likewise helps to repair skin damage and speed tissue healing. It's especially good to eat when you have a breakout.

BROCCOLI

Broccoli contains sky-high levels of vitamin C (the highest of all cruciferous vegetables), which is essential for the synthesis of collagen, the protein that gives structure to your skin. Broccoli also contains vitamins E and A, so it's a triple threat to oxidative aggressors that age the skin at a cellular level.

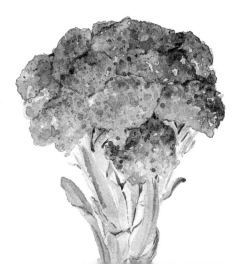

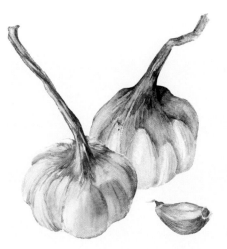

KALE, COLLARD GREENS AND SWISS CHARD

Vitamin A, which is found in these dark leafy greens, normalizes oil production so it's especially helpful for oily, acne-prone skin. These greens are all delicious and beneficial when incorporated into a broth-based soup.

BEETROOT AND BEET GREENS

Packed with folate, iron, fibre, potassium and manganese, these vibrant root vegetables add a unique earthiness to raw juices and salads. Beet greens (the top leafy part of the plant) are delicious in soups and with sautéed veggies. Beetroots are especially beneficial for women during their menstrual cycle and postpartum.

GARLIC

It's no wonder garlic is a staple ingredient in multicultural kitchens around the world. It contains a compound called allicin that helps to kill bacteria, reduce inflammation and improve circulation, and offers antioxidant benefits. There's nothing more comforting in the kitchen than the sound and smell of minced garlic simmering in warm olive oil.

FRUITS

Eat a rainbow! By loading up on fruits that represent the full spectrum of colour, you'll absorb a wide array of wholesome nutritional properties from your multicoloured plate. Fruits are generally high in fibre and loaded with vitamin C, which boosts collagen production and supports optimal adrenal function to help you better cope with the stresses of daily life at a cellular level.

AVOCADOS

There's a whole culture surrounding love for avocados; from fuzzy throw cushions to avocado-printed pyjamas, the avocado obsession runs deep. And for good reason! These beauty foods are packed with healthy omega fats, which nourish and hydrate skin from within. The antioxidants in avocados renew damaged skin cells, help retain moisture and benefit skin elasticity.

ACAI BERRIES

You may have seen acai bowls listed on the menu at your local smoothie shop. This exotic fruit from South America was recently dubbed a 'superfood', because the berries are rich in skin-protecting antioxidants, trace minerals, amino acids and electrolytes.

BLUEBERRIES

These tiny berries work wonders for the skin! They are notably high in antioxidants, which are essential for reversing the effects of oxidative damage from our environment.

COCONUT

We all know about the glow-inducing benefits of minimally processed coconut oil applied topically (see a simple

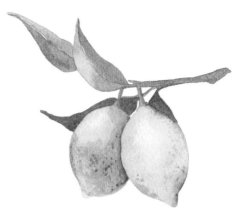

whipped body butter recipe on page 148), so it's no surprise the delicious meat is equally valuable. Fresh, young coconut meat contains B vitamins, potassium, amino acids, fibre, and live enzymes which help to boost immunity and bathe your skin with micronutrients from the inside out.

LEMONS

Warm water with lemon is one of the best ways to start your day! Lemons are high in vitamin C, which helps boost and strengthen collagen production and also works to neutralize excess acid in the body. The minerals found in lemons create more alkalinity, which can help soothe irritated skin, improve digestive health and fortify your immune system.

PINK AND RED GRAPEFRUIT

This breakfast staple is a brilliant beauty food and makes for a tangy, energizing start to your day. Red and pink grapefruit varieties get their gorgeous coral hue from carotenoids, which help to brighten skin tone and boost skin's elasticity.

RED GRAPES

Resveratrol, a plant polyphenol found in the skin of red grapes, is a powerful antioxidant, thought to protect against the sun's UV radiation and thus a skincare industry buzzword. You may have seen it listed as the cornerstone ingredient in many popular skincare lines. With a relatively low glycemic-index score, red grapes are a delicious way to eat this glow food straight from the source.

ESSENTIAL FATTY ACIDS

Essential fatty acids, such as omega-3 and omega-6, are powerful anti-inflammatory glow foods that moisturize your skin from the inside out.

CHIA SEEDS

Can you believe that this tiny-but-mighty speck of a seed contains more omega-3 in a single serving than salmon, and more antioxidants than blueberries? They're also an excellent source of protein and can help sustain your energy levels, which makes chia seeds a great mid-afternoon snack.

FLAXSEEDS

Used since ancient times for their mild nutty flavour and health benefits, flaxseeds are a delightful way to incorporate more fibre and skin-moisturizing omega-3 fatty acids into your diet. Add flaxseeds to homemade bread, muffins, granola and smoothies — or sprinkle over avocado toast or porridge with fresh berries.

OLIVE OIL

Extra virgin olive oil is a cultural staple that has been around for thousands of years. It's rich in oleic acid (an omega-9 fatty acid) and polyphenols, which help to hydrate skin and provide antioxidant support.

WALNUTS AND ALMONDS

These are great omega-rich beauty food snack options, both for their versatility and portability. Add walnuts to a salad or keep a stash of almonds at your desk for when hunger strikes. Lightly salted versions are a crunchy, satisfying alternative to processed crisps and crackers.

BEAUTY BOOSTERS

TURMERIC

This ancient golden root is a skin hero. It's packed with a bioactive compound called curcumin, which reduces inflammation, evens skin tone and speeds wound healing. It's a great addition for those working to heal atopic dermatitis, eczema and psoriasis.

CINNAMON

This warming spice contains potent antioxidants called polyphenols and flavonoids, which help to heal skin at the cellular level. Cinnamon is also a natural anti-inflammatory ingredient and boosts circulation for a healthy, rosy glow.

GINGER

Ginger is an all-star anti-inflammatory and invigorates the senses when taken internally or applied topically. It can also help with digestion and calm an upset stomach. I love adding fresh root ginger to blended smoothies and raw juices for an energizing burst of flavour.

PROBIOTICS AND PREBIOTICS

This synergistic duo help to rebalance the good bacteria in your digestive system – they nourish your gut on the inside, so that you'll glow on the outside! Fermented food and drinks, such as kombucha, kefir, kimchi and sauerkraut, are rich in probiotics. Onions, leeks, asparagus and garlic are all good sources of prebiotics.

DANDELION GREENS

You may have spotted dandelions in a field of wild flowers or, perhaps, popping up as a pesky weed in your garden, but you might be surprised to know that this humble plant has powerful medicinal properties that have been utilized in traditional remedies for centuries. Brewed tea made from dandelion leaves boasts skin health benefits and helps aid in efficient digestion. You can also explore culinary uses for the root and flower, which are both edible.

THE GUT-GLOW CONNECTION:
PLANT-POWERED BEAUTY ELIXIRS

Gut-friendly and glow-inducing, these beauty beverage recipes are filled with plant-based ingredients to keep your skin healthy. They're delicious, too!

HOMEMADE CASHEW MILK

This is my all-time favourite milk to make at home, because it requires no straining! If you've ever tried making your own almond milk, you'll know that straining it can be a time-consuming extra step, so cashew milk is a simple alternative that is delectably rich and creamy. I use this as a base for cashew ice cream, to top granola, in smoothies and beyond… It's delicious and loaded with skin-loving minerals such as selenium, magnesium and zinc.

MAKES 1 LITRE (34 FL OZ)
125g (4½oz/1 cup) raw cashew nuts | 1 litre (1¾ pints/4 cups) water
pinch of sea salt | 2 pitted dates (optional)

Soak the raw cashew nuts in a covered bowl of water overnight.

The next day, drain off and discard the soaking liquid. Place the soaked cashews in a high-speed blender, along with the measured fresh water and sea salt, then blend for 1 minute. You can also add a couple of pitted dates to the blender, if you want a touch of sweetness.

Store covered in the refrigerator for up to three days.

NO-MILK HOT COCOA WITH COLLAGEN

There's something nostalgic about a steaming cup of hot cocoa on a chilly winter night. This beauty beverage will give you the holiday warm-and-fuzzies without tons of added sugar or dairy. Organic raw cacao is considered a beauty food because it is high in iron, magnesium and calcium. Plus, you can add a scoop of your favourite collagen powder to boost the benefits! If you'd prefer a refreshing smoothie to a warm drink, add the ingredients to a blender with half a frozen banana and blitz into a scrumptious smoothie.

SERVES 1

225ml (8fl oz/1 cup) cashew milk (homemade is best!)
1½ teaspoons raw cacao powder │ 2.5cm (1in) square of plain dark chocolate
5 drops of vanilla extract │ 1 scoop collagen powder (use the scoop
that comes in the pack or the recommended dose)
pinch each of cinnamon and sea salt, to serve

Combine all the ingredients in a saucepan and gently warm through. Use a whisk to blend the cacao powder and melted chocolate to a frothy, smooth consistency. Pour into a mug and top with a pinch each of cinnamon and sea salt.

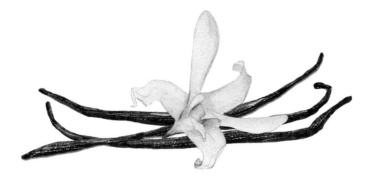

ICED MATCHA GREEN TEA

The matcha mania is real. And, luckily for your skin, it's *real* good! Matcha is packed with specific antioxidants called polyphenols, which fight free-radical damage and inflammation. It is also rich in vitamins, minerals and amino acids, which will add a micronutrient infusion to your morning pick-me-up. You may have tried green tea in the past, but matcha is in a league of its own. This bright-green beauty beverage is created with whole green tea leaves that are ground into a fine powder, so you will consume more of the plant goodness in each delicious sip. It originally came from China, where it was used by Zen monks who needed a burst of focus before entering long meditation sessions. Look for ceremonial-grade matcha powder that does not include sugar or other synthetic additives.

SERVES 1

½ teaspoon ceremonial-grade matcha powder
½ teaspoon coconut nectar or raw honey (optional)
60ml (2fl oz/¼ cup) hot water │ 3–4 ice cubes
175ml (6fl oz/¾ cup) almond milk

Combine the matcha and sweetener (if using) in a drinking vessel.
Pour over the hot water and use a whisk to dissolve the matcha.
Add the ice and almond milk, then stir to combine.

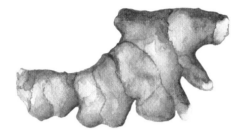

GINGER, LEMON AND APPLE CIDER VINEGAR TONIC

This easy-to-make tonic will fight inflammation, boost your immune system and aid digestion to keep you energized and glowing. The taste is pungent and may be bracing for some, so I suggest drinking it like a shot before your first meal of the day. You could also take it as a tea and sip throughout the day.

MAKES 8 SHOTS
450ml (16fl oz/2 cups) water
2.5cm (1 in) piece of fresh organic root ginger, peeled and diced
juice of ½ lemon │ 2 tablespoons apple cider vinegar

In a small saucepan, bring the water and ginger to the boil, then reduce the heat and simmer for 15 minutes to create an infused ginger tea. Add the fresh lemon juice and apple cider vinegar.

Alternatively, juice the fresh ginger in a juicer before combining with freshly boiled water and the other ingredients.

Enjoy warm or allow to cool, then store in an airtight container in the refrigerator for up to a week.

GOLDEN TURMERIC LATTE

This yummy latte alternative is like a cup of golden liquid sunshine. When cooking, I try to sprinkle in anti-inflammatory turmeric wherever I can (a pinch added to scrambled eggs; a dash on roasted cauliflower; a heaped tablespoon in vegetable soup), but to get the benefits of this beauty booster, my preferred way by far is to enjoy it in a foamy latte. Using fresh turmeric here really knocks it out of the park, but, if you don't have it, just swap for 1 teaspoon ground turmeric. The addition of black pepper allows your body to better absorb the curcumin from the turmeric.

SERVES 1

225ml (8fl oz/1 cup) full-fat coconut milk

1 teaspoon peeled and grated fresh turmeric | 1 teaspoon coconut oil

dash of sea salt and freshly ground black pepper

1 tablespoon coconut sugar, raw honey or maple syrup (optional)

Place all the ingredients into a saucepan set over a high heat and warm through, whisking until combined.

Alternatively, warm the coconut milk first, then add all the ingredients to a blender and blitz until smooth.

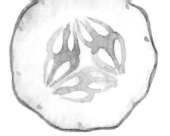

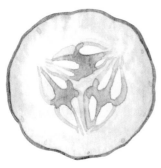

CUCUMBER LIME REFRESHER WITH CHIA SEEDS

When added to liquid, chia seeds form a gel-like coating around each individual seed. This offers a chance to enjoy a new sensory experience when drinking this beauty elixir and it also yields a major hydration pay-off. Chia seeds come from a desert plant and were intricately designed by nature to absorb and retain 30 times their own weight in water. This drink is especially refreshing on hot days when you're feeling sluggish and dehydrated.

SERVES 4

3 tablespoons chia seeds │ 700ml (1½ pints/3 cups) water
1 organic cucumber │ juice of 1 lime │ 1 tablespoon coconut nectar

Add the chia seeds to 225ml (8fl oz/1 cup) water, stir thoroughly, then cover and place in the refrigerator overnight.

The next day, blend the remaining 475ml (16fl oz/2 cups) water with the cucumber, lime juice and coconut nectar in a high-speed blender. Combine the chia water with the cucumber lime water and enjoy!

A TROUBLESOME TRIO

While they aren't an issue for everyone, gluten, sugar and dairy are the three foods that I often advise clients to eliminate from their diet for a time. Often, the impact of these foods is subtle. While you may not be allergic, you could have a sensitivity or intolerance that causes belly bloat and breakouts.

I suggest keeping a food journal for two weeks and commit to eating clean, organic whole foods. Writing down each bite tends to create a better sense of accountability and, therefore, yields better results. Listen to your body – especially after the two weeks have passed and you begin moderately reintroducing foods one at a time. You will be able to pinpoint which foods are causing breakouts, headaches, gas and other unpleasant symptoms. Once you identify the offending foods, you'll be able to avoid them.

GLUTEN

This sticky and difficult-to-digest protein has had a bad rap lately. Food companies will affix a 'gluten-free' label to everything these days – to the point of absurdity (in 2018, there was an article on BBC online about 'gluten-free', 'kosher' and 'organic' bottled water being marketed and sold at a premium!). There's no doubt that the gluten-free craze has gone too far; however, some of the hype may be founded. People with the auto-immune disorder coeliac disease can experience severe chronic inflammation and digestive issues. For some, it's simply a sensitivity that can cause abdominal pain and bloating. And fewer still are those who aren't necessarily sensitive to gluten, but due to an over-processed diet consume too much in too many foods too frequently. This excess can cause an inflammatory response in the body and exacerbate skin conditions such as psoriasis, eczema, acne and severely dry skin. For most people, occasional moderate amounts of gluten will not be a problem. When you next get a craving for a slice of buttered toast, I suggest eating fermented sourdough with clarified ghee butter.

SUGAR

Simple sugars are like an addictive drug. When you eat a sugary pastry or drink a bottle of soft drink (a 600ml (20oz) bottle contains the jaw-dropping equivalent of 17 teaspoons of sugar!), a large quantity of insulin is produced in a rapid effort to regulate the sudden overload of sugar in your bloodstream. This spike in sugar and insulin causes that fast-but-fleeting energy boost. The benefit is short-lived, because once your insulin level returns to normal, your body tells you it wants another rush and so the vicious cycle continues.

In addition, when you satisfy sugar cravings, your skin suffers. The rapid rise of blood-sugar levels causes a reaction in the cells called glycation. This takes place when sugar molecules adhere and bond themselves to the skin's collagen and cause this structural protein to become malformed. This weakens the skin's ability to maintain healthy structure and form. Often skin is less 'springy' or 'bouncy' because the elastin has been damaged and will show fine lines, wrinkles and loss of radiance. Excess sugar intake is one of the fastest ways to age your skin. If you've already done some damage, you can help rebuild collagen with facial treatments such as micro-needling collagen induction therapy and red light LED sessions, and by drinking lots of green tea, which is known to boost collagen production.

DAIRY

Dairy is the last of the troublesome trio. There are some cases when dairy is considered a health food (think: small amounts of organic cultured butter and full-fat yogurt), but most often it's consumed as a processed food in sweetened yogurts, ice cream and cheeses. Lactose and the casein protein found in dairy products are both responsible for triggering belly bloating, brain fog, sinus congestion, eczema, acne and gas.

In addition, the consumption of dairy could potentially trigger and contribute to acne and skin inflammation. That's because the majority of milk produced in commercial dairies comes from cows that are continually impregnated so that they will keep lactating. These hormones are passed on to us through the milk and may play a role in generating excess sebum production, which often ignites acne. Excess sebum production and cystic acne, especially around the chin, jawline and neck, are influenced by androgens and growth-factor hormones found in milk and other animal by-products. If we think for a moment about the absurdity of the fact that humans are the only mammals to drink milk after infancy, and that the milk from a lactating cow is different in composition from what best nourishes our unique human bodies, it becomes easier to see why ditching dairy may be a good choice.

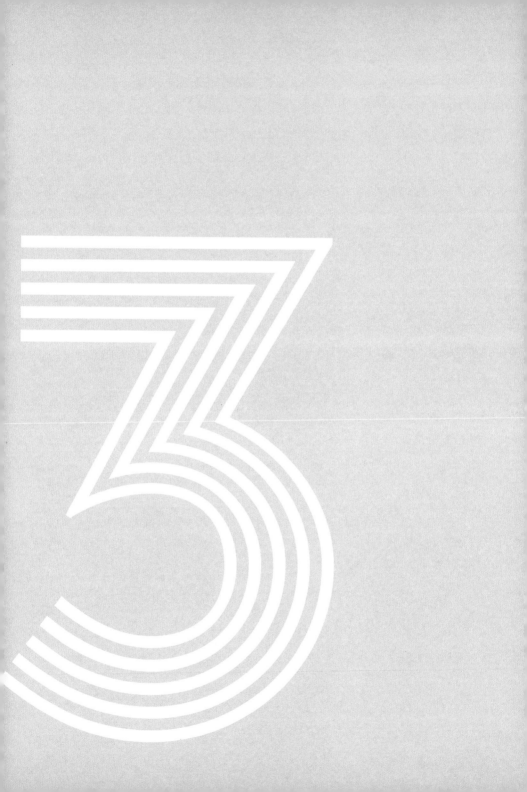

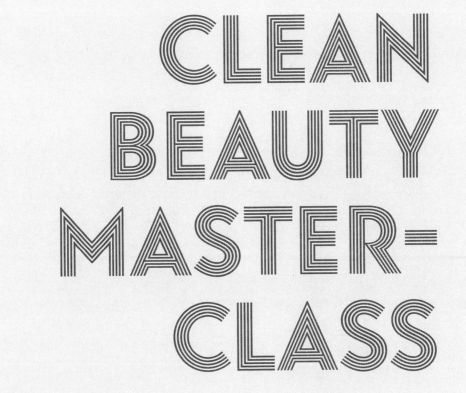

CLEAN
BEAUTY
MASTER-
CLASS

SKINCARE FOR SELF-CARE

Do you view your skincare as a practice, in the same way that meditation, exercise or a hobby is a practice? Or is your skincare routine an automatic hygiene obligation that daunts you at the end of each day? Many of my clients, like most people, find themselves in the second category. Maybe it's because you're feeling over-extended in life and washing your face feels like one more repetitious requirement on your to-do list. Or maybe you want to enjoy your skincare, but feel utterly paralyzed by the options and aren't sure how to find what's right for your unique skin type.

I invite you to throw all of those feelings out of the window and imagine your skincare as a ritual, not a routine – a pleasurable sensory experience that you will look forward to. Doesn't that sound amazing? Remember this: *self-care is not selfish*. When you prioritize your personal wellness, you will end up with an abundance of energy to give generously to your family, friends, career and the world. Can you commit to carving out a non-negotiable space, especially in the midst of a busy or challenging day, for a brief moment of self-care that is altogether yours?

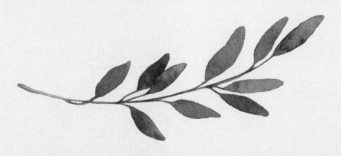

BUILDING YOUR SKINCARE RITUAL

You've probably been there: standing perplexed in front of a shelf filled with a seemingly unending array of products from various brands. In this age of excess, how does one choose exactly what's needed? Becoming familiar with the role of each product type will help you better understand what your skin needs, plus when and how to use it.

There are times when simply swapping your cleanser can be a complete game changer for your skin. Or, perhaps, you're accidently sabotaging your skin by using an astringent when your skin is really longing for a hydrating toning mist. The world of skincare is wide and companies are always coming up with new ways to say the same old thing. And even for a savvy skincare shopper, all of the products available can be baffling. Here, you'll learn the lowdown about the different products available and how they impact your skin. I'll also unpack the answers to the most commonly asked questions, compiled from years working one-on-one with clients in the treatment room.

THE FACIAL CLEANSER

Cleansing is the first step in any skincare lineup. A good facial cleanser should thoroughly refresh skin without disrupting its natural protective oil and water barrier. Cleansers detoxify the skin and remove surface impurities such as dirt, sebum, sweat, pollution, bacteria and dead skin cell build-up. These environmental elements, which skin comes into contact with daily, obstruct the proper penetration of active plant compounds. That means, applying topical antioxidants and nourishing phytochemicals will not be as effective if the skin is bogged down with congestion and micro-toxins in the pores. This is why cleansing is a vitally important step, and finding the right cleanser is key to supporting long-term skin wellness.

THE LOWDOWN ON CLEANSER TYPES

CLEANSING OIL/BALM Basic cosmetic chemistry teaches that 'like attracts like', meaning oil attracts oil, which is why these cleansers are the best for deeply cleaning skin without the use of harsh foaming detergents that disrupt your natural protective barrier. Facial cleansing oils are one of life's simple luxuries. Whether you're using it as a pre-cleansing make-up remover, or as your standalone cleanser, oils swish away make-up, dirt and oil in every skin type. If your skin feels tight, dry and irritated, no matter how much moisture you apply, try oil cleansing. Over time, it will allow your body to repair its natural barrier function that may have been compromised, and your skin will become softer and calmer.

The one drawback I often hear from clients is that they feel as though the oil is just sitting on the surface of the skin. To solve this, I always recommend using a soft face cloth or a facial chamois (or 'shammy' – an extra-soft flannel). Dampen the cloth under warm water and use it to compress the skin, then remove the cleanser in gentle circular motions.

Sometimes, you'll see cleansing oils in balm form. Cleansing balms or balm sticks are another way to formulate oil-based ingredients and can be used in the same way with a warm soft washcloth.

CLEANSING CREAM/LOTION Creamy cleansers are formulated with oils and moisturizing compounds, which dissolve make-up, dirt and epidermal debris to clean skin without stripping away your natural protective barrier. You'll also see them referred to as cleansing milk or cleansing lotion. Usually suggested for dry, sensitive skin types, cleansing creams make skin feel soft. Since these usually don't rely on surfactants to lift away impurities, cream cleansers can't always be trusted to remove heavier make-up and sunscreen. In this case, pre-cleanse with oil, and then use the cream cleanser as a quick second cleanse to ensure you aren't leaving any residue behind.

CLEANSING GEL Gel or foam cleansers are often formulated to 'degrease' the skin and whisk away every trace of natural sebum on the skin surface. For someone with oily skin, or who is experiencing minor breakouts, it's tempting to think gel cleansers are the answer, when actually they could be making the issue worse. These formulas are typically clear in colour and often contain other clarifying

Q & A: DO I NEED TO CLEANSE SKIN MORNING AND NIGHT?

Sometimes, it can feel redundant to cleanse your skin in the morning when you went to bed with clean skin from washing the night before, right? However, overnight is when your skin repairs and restores itself. In the process, it often secretes sebum and flushes toxin build-up. There's also the little issue of drool. It's possible that you're introducing inevitable bacteria to your skin and pillowcase from unknowingly sleeping with your mouth agape. Cleansing after sleeping removes all of the above – oil, bacteria and heavier nighttime products – to give you a fresh canvas that will drink up the fresh nutrients that you apply in the morning.

ingredients, such as tea tree oil, witch hazel and benzoyl peroxide. There are occasions – and very specific skin types – that I believe benefit from using cleansing gel; however, I would rarely suggest it be used twice daily. You may consider using a gel cleanser two or three times per week to clarify skin. If you are experiencing acne or overly oily skin, I encourage you to try cleansing oils used with a soft washcloth, rather than consistently stripping skin of natural moisture, which encourages your body to overproduce more oil in an effort to replace what's being removed each day.

THE EXFOLIATOR

Exfoliators essentially remove the outermost layer of dead epidermal cells on the surface of your skin. This helps with skin texture and also encourages the lower layers of your skin to produce new, fresh skin cells (through a process called 'cellular turnover'). When the top dead cells are swept away, this allows your skincare to penetrate more deeply for better results. Your skin does naturally shed dead skin cells, and will do so without any extra help, however this biological process slows down with age, so boosting your skin's natural abilities will assist your skin in functioning more optimally.

Often my clients fall into two categories: those who rarely exfoliate, and those who exfoliate obsessively. If you're somewhere in between then you're already one step ahead and on the way to a healthy skincare routine! Exfoliating twice a week is recommended as a general rule. Over-exfoliating could be the biggest mistake for your skin. Between never exfoliating and over-exfoliating, I believe the latter has the most detrimental impact on your skin. In the past, I've heard clients say, 'I love the burn – if it's stinging, it *must* be working!' But the truth is that almost every negative symptom of the skin can be connected to an imbalanced or damaged 'barrier function'.

Your skin barrier is the outermost layer of skin called the *stratum corneum*, a mix of natural oils and a microcosm of beneficial bacteria, which protects you from the environment, defends against pathogenic bacteria via a slight natural acidity, helps retain water moisture and keeps skin looking radiant. When you over-do it with exfoliants, tiny cracks form in your skin's barrier, which allow bacteria in and moisture to invariably seep out. This can be seen in the form of dehydration, dryness, increased sensitivity, breakouts, redness, peeling, rough skin texture and general inflammation. When you continually strip the skin barrier with high-foam surfactants, drying acne ingredients, astringents and exfoliants, you can bet that eventually your skin will feel tight, dry and irritated.

THE LOWDOWN ON EXFOLIATORS

When it comes to exfoliation, there are two types to consider: physical and chemical. Physical exfoliation refers to the use of anything that physically abrades skin to buff away dead cellular build-up. Chemical exfoliation is the use of compounds to gently loosen and dissolve the sticky glue-like bonds between dead skin cells. Both are marvellous tools for skin health, and yet both can cause major skin damage if not used properly.

PHYSICAL EXFOLIATORS Some popular physical exfoliators include rotary spinning brushes, dry lymphatic facial brushes, konjac sponges, granular scrubs and washcloths. If you do choose to use a spinning cleansing brush, make sure to use the most gentle, soft bristles on the lowest, most gentle setting. Allow the brush to do the work for you; do not apply added pressure. If the bristles of your brush are splaying outwards and becoming misshapen, you are pressing too hard. Another consideration with rotary brushes is sanitation. Clean them often and don't store them in damp, dark or dirty places (that's the environment where bacteria thrive!).

Another topic that often comes up with clients is the type of granule used in a scrub. There are thousands of facial scrubs on the

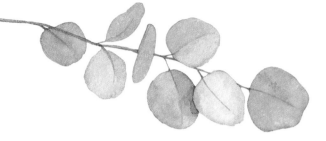

market and not all are created equal. Avoid anything with a large granular size, even if they are naturally derived, such as ground nut shells or fruit pits. These are often sharp (even if you can't see it with the naked eye) and cause micro-lacerations on the surface of the skin. This causes unnecessary inflammation and allows germs to enter the skin more easily. Often, I advise a granular scrub that is in a fine powder form. The texture should be soft, never scratchy.

In professional spa treatments, two popular types of physical exfoliation are dermaplaning and microdermabrasion.

CHEMICAL EXFOLIATORS

Chemical exfoliants can be naturally derived or synthetic. They often contain alpha hydroxy acid (AHA), beta hydroxy acid (BHA), enzymes, or a blend of all three. In professional treatments, chemical exfoliators can range anywhere from intense, heavy-duty medical-grade peels to super-gentle fruit-based enzymes that barely penetrate the top layers of the skin. Often chemical peels are misused and over-used even by skincare professionals with the best intentions.

THE TONER

Facial toners are fast-absorbing liquid products that restore skin's pH balance, deliver anti-inflammatory ingredients, hydrate and sweep away impurities that your cleanser may have missed. In addition, toner preps your skin to readily absorb oil and moisturizers. A good analogy is to think of your skin as a sponge. Imagine pouring oil onto a completely dry, stiff sponge. It would likely drip right off and not be absorbed much at all. Then imagine the same oil poured onto a wet sponge. It's much more likely to absorb the oil, because it has been prepped and softened. Your skin is similar, in that it needs water and oil to be most happy and healthy. That's why layering facial oils onto skin while it's still damp with toner will result in deeper penetration and much more moisture.

Toners are applied after cleansing, but before applying moisturizer. Treatment toners, which contain exfoliating ingredients like salicylic or glycolic acid, are best applied with a cotton wool ball or pad, whereas essences and hydrosol mists can be applied or spritzed directly onto the face, with the option to softly pat the skin until the toner is absorbed. As a general guideline, you have about three minutes to tone and moisturize from the time you get out of the shower or bath. Aiming to apply products within this window of time will help you to seal in moisture while your skin is still damp.

THE LOWDOWN ON TONERS

FACIAL MIST For home care, I suggest opting for fruit enzymes, which gently encourage cell turnover with little risk of causing an inflammatory response. Enzymes break down the keratinized protein found in the outer layer of the epidermis, which incites skin to regenerate. Popular enzymes are pineapple, papaya, pumpkin and tart cherries. Natural AHA alternatives, such as yogurt (which contains lactic acid), sugar (which contains glycolic acid) and grapes (which contain tartaric acid), are great options for DIY preparations.

Facial toning mists typically contain hydrosols, a type of botanical water made from herbs or flowers. Hydrosols are created during the steam distillation process of making essential oils. During distillation, the essential oil is separated from the water, which leaves behind an infused water that still retains the properties of the plant from which it was extracted. These waters are much more diluted than essential oils themselves and can be used liberally many times throughout the day. Some of the most popular hydrosols are rose, lavender, tea tree, neroli, calendula, lemongrass and sage. If dewy, hydrated skin is your goal, these should be your go-to products. Somehow, there are still skincare professionals who consider toning mists to be superfluous, but from my experience they are one of the fundamental steps in any great skincare routine.

Mist onto clean skin immediately before applying face oil. *It's really important not to let the toner completely dry on your skin before applying your serum or oil.* When you apply the two together, your skin drinks up the nutrients and saturates your cells in water and oil moisture for deep hydration. You can also mist on top of make-up and sunscreen throughout the day, whenever your skin feels dehydrated. Whether you're standing in front of your bathroom mirror, at your desk, out on the beach or scrunched on a stagnant aeroplane, one spritz of a herbal face mist immediately refreshes your skin and creates an uplifting moment of aromatherapy.

ASTRINGENT OR TREATMENT TONER

Treatment toners often contain a cocktail of exfoliating enzymes or alpha-hydroxy acids, like lactic acid or glycolic acid, to dissolve the build-up of dead skin cells. Some treatment toners also contain fermented ingredients, such as probiotics or kombucha tea, to balance skin's natural surface micro-flora.

Astringents are often marketed to oily, acne-prone skin types because they typically contain alcohol, which has a drying effect on the skin. It seems clients with oilier skin love this tight, dry sensation because it gives the illusory feeling of smaller pores and squeaky-clean skin. However, in reality, it's just dehydrating the skin and disrupting your body's natural barrier. As a general rule, I don't recommend harsh astringents and wince if a client tells me they've been using isopropyl alcohol on their skin as a toner. Witch hazel is a nice natural alternative to astringents, which balances and clarifies skin without over-stripping it.

ESSENCE Facial essences emerged into the mainstream skincare scene when Korean or 'K-Beauty' increased in popularity. These are similar to a toner but are infused with a serum, which gives the product a more slippery, gel-like consistency. In Korean beauty rituals, essences are applied in multiple layers and then gently tapped or patted into the skin in order for the nutrients to penetrate. Some essences contain hyaluronic acid, a moisture-binding humectant that is great for hydrating skin.

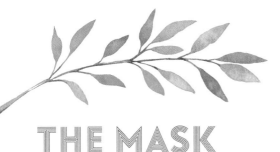

THE MASK

Consider masks to be a supplemental step in your skincare ritual. Facial masks are typically applied onto the skin in a thick layer to deliver antioxidants, soothe irritation, clarify oil and refine skin, then are rinsed with water or removed with a warm towel. There are many different types available, from hydrating creamy textures to sheet masks, powdered clay or mineral mud masks.

Masks add value because they are targeted treatments used for varying skin conditions. Most directions will instruct leaving the product on for 15–20 minutes, which means using them can be a candle-lit luxurious experience, or they can be worn while multi-tasking. Tackling a sinkful of dishes suddenly becomes more enjoyable when your skin is coated in aromatic, skin-healing antioxidants.

THE LOWDOWN ON MASKS

HYDRATING MASKS Delivered in the form of ultra-rich creams, gels and sheet masks, these products are meant to infuse dry skin with moisture. Plant-based hydrating masks include ingredients like avocado, royal jelly, water-dense fruits, aloe vera and vegetable glycerine.

CLARIFYING MASKS Typically formulated with clay or mud, these masks are oil-absorbing and work to draw impurities out of the skin. Natural clarifying mask ingredients include kaolin white clay, charcoal and marine clay, as well as botanicals such as chamomile, dandelion root, lavender, lemon and tea tree, to clarify congested skin and calm breakouts.

BRIGHTENING MASKS These masks specifically treat pigmentation spots by targeting and regulating the enzyme that triggers an overproduction of melanin. Natural skin brighteners include vitamin C, kojic acid, bearberry leaf and liquorice root.

EXFOLIATING MASKS The purpose of an exfoliating mask is to eliminate dead skin build-up. They often contain acids such as glycolic, lactic, tartaric and salicylic, or any combination of fruit enzymes such as papaya, pineapple, pumpkin, cranberry and mango.

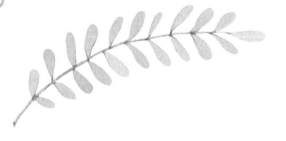

THE MOISTURIZER

Facial moisturizers provide a thin protective coating on the outermost layer of skin. Your skin inherently does this on its own by producing sebum, but, moisturizers enhance your body's natural function by delivering antioxidant-rich nutrients to hydrate the cells and helping to protect the skin from external environmental damage. Moisturizers also slow the process of transepidermal water loss, where water moisture evaporates from your skin into the surrounding atmosphere. Moisturizers can be delivered in the form of serums, facial oils, creams and balms. They are typically the last step in your skincare routine, excluding sun protection, and should be applied with upward massaging strokes or patted gently into the skin.

THE LOWDOWN ON MOISTURIZERS

SERUM Serums are formulated with ingredients that have the ability to penetrate beyond the surface to repair skin at a cellular level. Often, serums are marketed as being the most precious and highly concentrated free-radical-fighting products to counteract skin damage, and usually come with the highest price tag. Skincare companies know shoppers will shell out cash for the term 'serum'. Serums tend to have a thinner viscosity than most face oils and can sometimes feel like a gel or a very lightweight oil. Traditional serums are water-based; however, as the trend expands, more companies are referring to their face oil as serum.

AMPOULES Ampoules were popular in professional spa lines for years, but now are available to the public, especially in Korean skincare. Ampoules are serums packaged in small vials, designed to be opened fresh for single-use application. The idea is that, if serums truly do contain high concentrations of antioxidants, especially vitamin C, they are much less stable and prone to oxidation every time you open the bottle and expose the product to the air. Ampoules are a way to ensure the product remains potent up to the minute it is applied to your skin.

FACE OIL There isn't a skin type on the planet that doesn't benefit from face oil. For many years, oils were villainized as the bad guys – the pore-clogging, blackhead-causing ingredients to avoid. Perhaps that's true for a heavy mineral oil, but for a lightweight, nutrient-rich, plant-based oil it's not the case. Even the most oily, breakout-prone skin will benefit from a small amount of face oil because it helps to regulate skin's own natural sebum production. If you're consistently stripping the skin of all natural oils and applying a drying acne

Q & A: WHY ARE THESE CALLED 'ACTIVE' PRODUCTS?

That sounds as though they will irritate my skin. Often, we only hear of AHA (alpha hydroxy acid) and BHA (beta hydroxy acid) exfoliants being dubbed as 'active' products, but basically this term refers to the product in your beauty lineup that's causing the most *action* – the most change in the skin or the most results. And, yes, sometimes that may refer to a chemical AHA exfoliant or to retinol. But in fact, there are soothing, hydrating active plant compounds (such as green tea, ferulic acid, lycopene and many other whole plants) that will actively support and protect your skin. Everything you do in your skincare ritual up to this point – cleansing, exfoliating, toning – prepares your skin to readily absorb these powerful ingredients. Since most moisturizers are rich in antioxidants and vitamins, they tend to pack the most meaningful punch when it comes to treating skin conditions like hyperpigmentation, acne and rosacea.

product, like sulphur or benzoyl peroxide, the skin becomes confused and, in turn, produces more oil because that's how your body protects itself. Oils can be incredibly balancing and the antioxidants they deliver are an effective acne treatment.

Always use face oils with a toning mist. Press 3–4 drops onto skin that is still damp from a hydrosol toning mist and both will absorb deeply into your skin.

Stash a bottle of face oil in your bag and apply a few drops throughout the day. This is a refreshing midday pick-me-up, especially under the eyes, because moisturizing plant-based oil plumps the skin and makes your whole complexion look dewy in an instant.

FACE CREAM Face creams are known to combat dehydration and restore radiance to parched skin; however, they aren't always necessary. Any great moisturizing cream contains an emulsion of water and oil, but the trick is getting these two ingredients to coexist. Naturally, they want to repel one another and eventually the product will separate causing the oil to float on top of the water. Cosmetic chemists work hard to find ways to bind these two ingredients together, and often end up using unneeded ingredients that benefit the texture without adding any meaningful value to the skin. The best way to achieve the benefits of a cream without all of the extra ingredients is to use a water-based hydrosol toning mist mixed with a natural plant oil. Combining the two directly on the skin offers your cells the water moisture they crave and the defending surface oil that the skin needs – all in one quick step.

BALM Facial balms are waterless oil-based products that replenish oil and act as a protective barrier for your skin. Balms create a layer on top of the skin to lock in moisture and protect you from the elements. They're especially beneficial in cooler winter months, or when skin is compromised and in need of healing. Some of my favourite facial balms contain rose, sandalwood and frankincense, which are intensely moisturizing and help soothe inflamed skin.

Q & A: IS AN EXTRA PRODUCT FOR EYES REALLY NECESSARY?

In order to treat it properly, it's important to understand how the skin around the eyes differs from the rest of the face. Our eyes are very expressive – we blink about 10,000 times per day, using 22 muscles that are in constant motion. Couple this with the fact that the skin around your eyes is the thinnest on your whole body (and does not contain oil glands or collagen fibres) and you've got a recipe for dehydrated skin and expression creases. So, yes! Using a product that is specifically formulated to replenish hydration and nurture this most delicate skin, while still being safe to apply around your sensitive eyes, will make a difference. For a DIY idea, see the Gentle Eye Serum recipe on page 125.

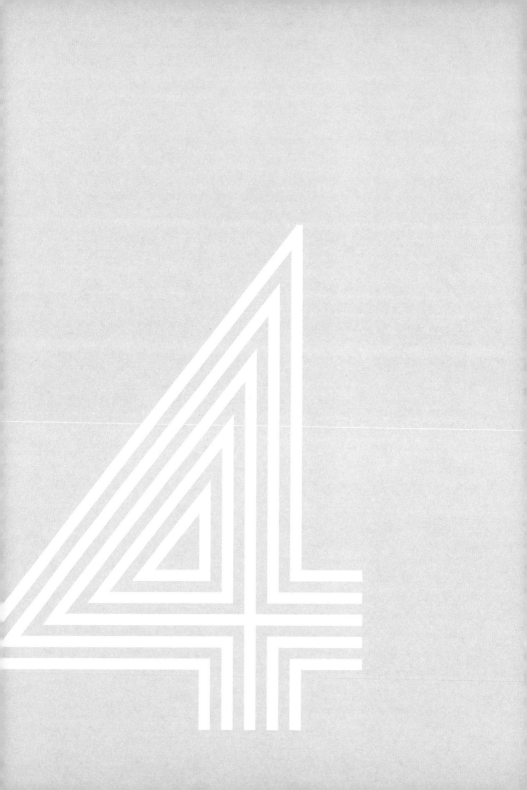

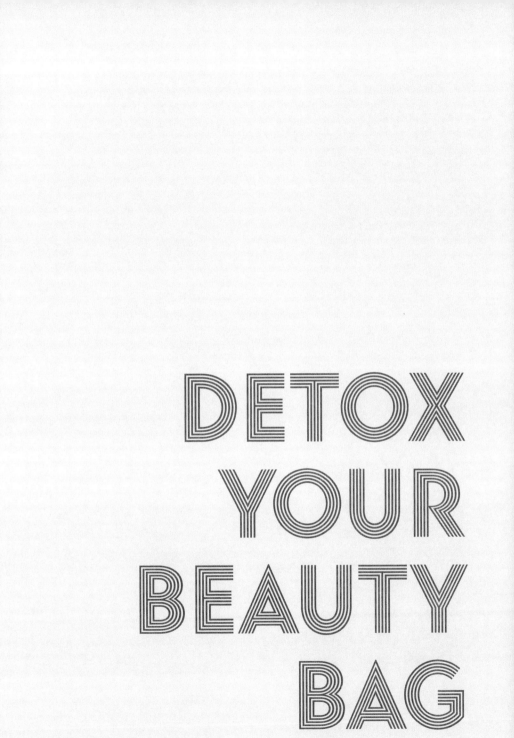

DETOX
YOUR
BEAUTY
BAG

HOW TO CLEANSE YOUR BEAUTY ROUTINE

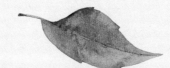

The organic, natural beauty market is booming. Brands with natural or botanically derived ingredients represent the largest share of high-end skincare sales, valued in billions. More than ever, we are hyper-aware of what we put into and onto our bodies and, as a result, we are demanding more transparency from beauty brands. This is such an exciting time to clean your beauty routine! Using plant-based skincare allows you to align your outer appearance with your inner beliefs for overall wellness. It's also a chance to use purchase-power to support brands that empower their employees and care for the environment.

Think about this: if our lives are the reflection of our actions and beliefs, then each time we make the choice to purchase another product, we are voting for that product – for the manufacturing methods, for the ingredients, for the packaging. We're placing our trust in that skincare company. When examining and revamping your beauty bag, take a look at every aspect of the products that you welcome into your home. In addition to the purity of the product, other factors may play a role in your decision to purchase with intention. As you build your own unique plant-based beauty routine, consider these questions:

IS THE PACKAGING RECYCLABLE OR BIODEGRADABLE?

ARE THE PRODUCTS CRUELTY-FREE?

WHO FOUNDED THE LINE?

ARE THE INGREDIENTS SUSTAINABLY SOURCED OR WILD-HARVESTED?

DOES THE COMPANY GIVE ANY PORTION OF PROCEEDS TO CHARITY?

Cleaning your routine is an orientation towards a more intentional lifestyle. Creating your own personal set of standards will help to guide you to the products that are just right for you.

Here's a fun exercise: count up how many personal care products you use on a daily basis. Think about your make-up, dental, skincare and hair products. What's your number? Based on a survey done by the Environmental Working Group, the average woman uses at least 12 products each day. (I have to admit that there was a time when my daily product number was significantly higher than 12!) The study found that 12.2 million adults are exposing their bodies every day to ingredients that are known or probable carcinogens, via their personal care products. Some of these ingredients are endocrine disruptors, which is especially hazardous for women. Beauty products should not create a compounded toxic build-up or 'burden' in our bodies.

HOW TO READ INGREDIENT LABELS

It's important to understand how to read an ingredient label to know exactly what you're putting into your body. This little bit of know-how will save you time and money. You'll be able to skim quickly through an ingredients list like a pro, and know when to bypass products that market a few key buzz-word ingredients, only to find them buried at the bottom of the ingredients list and hardly present in the formula at all!

Order matters – especially when it comes to deciphering skincare ingredient labels. Each list, or 'deck', is compiled by order of concentration. The most highly concentrated ingredients are listed first and everything that follows is listed in descending order. If, for example, a product claims to be packed with antioxidant rich green tea, and you look at the label to see camellia sinensis leaf extract (green tea) listed at the bottom of the list (likely alongside fragrance and parabens), then you know that there isn't much of this ingredient found in the product at all. This was the active antioxidant ingredient that drew you to the product in the first place, but there's not enough concentration to justify the misleading marketing.

Another ingredient you'll often see is water. It is usually the first 'base ingredient' in conventional skincare. Sometimes, water makes up as much as 80 per cent of the formula! My experience with products that contain mostly water is that they don't last as long because they are much more diluted. The water does not hydrate your skin in the same way that drinking a glass of water does your cells. Most of the water evaporates from your skin a few minutes after application, leaving your skin still craving moisture. What's worse is that, typically, many more non-essential filler ingredients (think: fragrances, emulsifiers, alcohols) must be added to keep the product shelf-stable while still achieving a nice smooth texture.

It's important to note that natural plant compounds can still look like tongue-twisting ingredients when they are declared on labels under the chemical or Latin name. For example, a label may state 'dipotassium glycyrrhizate', which looks hard to pronounce and potentially toxic, but it's actually liquorice root extract, which is plant-based, brightening and beneficial. When you're researching a plant-based product, complicated ingredient extract names are typically the exception; in general, labels become much easier to understand. Often, plant-based beauty does not contain water; instead, the first ingredients are natural plant oils such as sweet almond, rosehip, jojoba, red raspberry seed, pumpkin seed and carrot seed. You'll also see plant butters such as shea and cocoa, and hardening agents like beeswax and candelilla wax, followed by essential oils. For the most therapeutic benefits, look for products that contain only genuine plant ingredients.

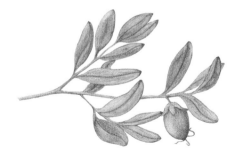

BEAUTY BLACKLIST

TOP 10 TOXIC INGREDIENTS TO AVOID

The simple truth that beauty companies don't want you to believe: you do not need hundreds of skincare and make-up products to achieve healthy skin.

Instead, you need a few (you can count them on one hand) hardworking, plant-based products to cleanse and renew skin and deliver antioxidant protection to your cells. Before we dive into what ingredients your skin is actually craving, let's go over the eyebrow-raising questionable ingredients to purge from your beauty routine, *forever*.

When it comes to cleaning your beauty products, focus on progress not perfection. This is my personal list of the top ten ingredients that I won't let into my beauty bag. There are so many innovative clean beauty alternatives on the market, you can say goodbye to these and never look back.

1 FRAGRANCE (Parfum, Perfume)

The main function of fragrances is to make the product smell appealing and they can be found across a wide array of products, from deodorant to mascara. Fragrance blends are often made up of a cocktail of toxic chemicals associated with neurotoxicity and hormone disruption, as well as eye, skin and respiratory irritation. An article published by the *Washington Post* called fragrance 'the new secondhand smoke' and quoted the Environmental Protection Agency saying that, because of the overuse of synthetic fragrance, our homes and work environments 'can be more seriously polluted than the outdoor air in even the largest and most industrialized cities'.

In New York, I worked at a spa in SoHo that specialized in fragrance- and allergen-free products for extremely sensitive customers. Clients would often come in looking exhausted and discouraged, with the results of their allergen patch test in hand. The ingredient that was almost ALWAYS at the top of the list to avoid was fragrance blends. 'But it's in *everything*,' they'd say to me, feeling completely overwhelmed. While these customers are an extreme example of how contact dermatitis can be impacted by synthetic fragrance, it's still wise to avoid this unnecessary toxic ingredient, even if you aren't specifically allergic.

2 CHEMICAL SUNSCREENS (Avobenzone, Oxybenzone, Homosalate, Benzophenone, Octisalate, Octinoxate)
The main function of these ingredients is to protect from the sun, but not all SPF is created equal. These 'chemical' ingredients (as opposed to mineral SPFs like zinc oxide or titanium dioxide) are known skin irritants and endocrine disruptors. Some of these sunscreen ingredients have been shown to cause damage to the oceans by destroying coral reefs. One study published by Environmental Health Perspectives estimates that up to 14,000 tons of sunscreen accumulates in the oceans globally each year. Instead, always opt for mineral sunscreen.

3 PARABENS (Methylparaben, Propylparaben, Isobutylparaben, Butylparaben)
At this point it feels a little clichéd to even talk about parabens. Most people have heard of these preservatives and have known for a while now that they aren't on the nice list. You'll see many companies promoting their products as 'paraben-free' and this certainly is progress. It's also a great example of how purchase-power moves the market. If we demand better products, companies will eventually deliver. Parabens are mostly an issue because, like fragrance, they are found everywhere. When you consider the compounded daily use of applying many products that contain these same preservatives, the amount becomes unsafe. Parabens mimic oestrogen and the Environmental Working Group reports that parabens have been found in human breast tissue.

4 SLS AND SLES (Sodium lauryl sulfate, Sodium laureth sulfate)
If it bubbles into a foamy lather, you can bet it contains either SLS or
SLES – cheap surfactant additives that leave everything from your
skin to your hair, clothes and teeth feeling 'squeaky clean'. These
should be blacklisted for this principle alone. The truth is that your skin
doesn't need to be stripped each day by these suds. In fact, this daily
use weakens skin's resilience and damages the natural protective
barrier function, which keeps you safe by protecting from bacterial
invaders. These ingredients are known to cause skin, eye and
respiratory irritation.

**5 MINERAL OIL AND PETROLEUM-DERIVED
INGREDIENTS**
Not only are these environmentally unkind, they also aren't great for
your skin. Mineral oils and petroleum jelly tend to be heavy, pore-
clogging moisturizers that block proper detoxification of the skin. They
form a water-tight barrier on top of the skin that can cause breakouts
in the acne-prone. Most skincare formulators like mineral oil because
it is inert, meaning it won't cause an allergic reaction, even though it
brings little therapeutic value to the product.

6 PHTHALATES (Dibutyl, Diethylhexyl and Diethyl phthalates)
Usually listed in the same breath with parabens, most phthalates have
been eliminated from many personal care products already, but it's still
good to be on the lookout. Phthalates help fragrance adhere to your
skin and are used to create a specific product texture. Phthalates are
endocrine disruptors and associated with birth defects. On the label,
look for dibutyl, diethylhexyl and diethyl phthalates.

7 HYDROQUINONE
Hydroquinone ranks high on the Environmental Working Group hazard
list. It's used to lighten skin and fade hyperpigmentation; however, the
risks far outweigh the benefits. Already banned in Australia, the
European Union and Japan, this ingredient raises concern around
cancer, organ toxicity, and skin and eye irritations. In some rare cases it
causes a blue-black coloured skin pigmentation called ocronosis when

over-the-counter formulas are used for an extended period of time. For brightening hyperpigmentation caused by inflammation, sun damage or hormones, choose plant-based ingredients like bearberry, kojic acid, mulberry, ferulic acid, white truffle, liquorice and carrot seed oil.

8 ALUMINIUM-BASED ANTIPERSPIRANT INGREDIENTS

Chemicals such as aluminium chlorohydrate and aluminium zirconium tetrachlorohydrex gly literally plug your sweat ducts so that you won't perspire. However, sweating is an important, sophisticated function your body uses to regulate temperature, purge toxins and ultimately keep you healthy. Alternatively, natural deodorants do not act as antiperspirants, but rather curb body odour by killing stink-causing bacteria via plant compounds, and absorbing wetness using ingredients like cornstarch or arrowroot powder. For a clean beauty bag, always opt for deodorant over antiperspirant.

9 TRICLOSAN

This anti-bacterial ingredient is found everywhere from your hand soap to laundry detergent or toothpaste. There's an ongoing debate about triclosan's safety and emerging research suggests that it may disrupt hormones as well as encourage the growth of drug-resistant bacteria. To make matters worse, triclosan has an environmental downside because it accumulates in lakes and streams.

10 TOULENE

Often found in nail polish and hair dyes, this ingredient is especially harmful for nail technicians and hair stylists who are exposed over a lifetime. However, those with auto-immune disorders, women who are pregnant and children should avoid it altogether. Most people report headaches, dizziness and skin irritation.

TOP 10 FAVOURITE PLANT-BASED INGREDIENTS

Now that you know what synthetic ingredients to ban from your beauty ritual, let's shine the spotlight onto the top ten plant-based ingredients. These are the tried-and-true ingredients I love and depend on the most – in the treatment room and for my own skin, too.

Thanks to our global marketplace, we now have access to thousands of natural raw materials, such as plant oils, extracts, powdered minerals, marine ingredients, essential oils and vitamins. It's empowering to have the know-how to create your own customised skincare, based on what your unique skin needs most. You'll learn more about how to use these and their benefits to skin in Chapter 7 (see page 90).

ALMOND FLOUR
(OR RICE BRAN POWDER)

Both act as a gentle facial scrub to remove impurities and micro-toxins from the pores. Rice bran is a by-product of rice milling and contains beneficial antioxidants. Skin looks bright and firm after using both these velvety-soft exfoliating ingredients. I love that they are customizable (you can add a small scoop to any cleanser or mask), extremely gentle even for the most reactive skin, and effectively decongest skin without causing any unnecessary inflammation.

CARROT SEED OIL

Carrot seed oil is rich in antioxidants to offset free radical skin damage caused by pollution and environmental aggressors. It is a natural source of SPF to protect skin from UV damage and is very high in beta-carotene, vitamin C and vitamin E.

FRUIT ENZYMES

Enzymes found in fruits like papaya, pineapple, tart cherries and mango are both antiinflammatory and exfoliating. They break down the keratinized bonds between skin cells – a gentle chemical process that removes excess cell buildup to reveal healthy, fresh skin. Fruit enzymes are often activated by heat, so use an enzyme mask in a steamy shower or with a warm washcloth used as a compress. Enzymes also boost the absorption of all other skincare products.

GLYCERINE

An important tool in any DIY skincare enthusiast's beauty pantry, glycerine is soluble in water and provides gentle cleansing properties without stripping skin of moisture. Distilled from vegetable oils, this clear, odourless ingredient behaves like a powerful humectant, drawing moisture from the air to the skin's surface like a magnet. Always check the label to ensure it's not blended with other, synthetic ingredients.

HYDROSOL FLORAL WATERS

There's something transformative about the soft, subtle scent of floral hydrosols. They boost moisture in the skin and are a simple way to squeeze self-care into a busy day. These mists contain antioxidants and micronutrients to cool and reduce redness, and most importantly, prepare skin to fully absorb the benefits from oils, balms and creams.

JOJOBA

Jojoba oil is a go-to multipurpose oil because it closely mimics your skin's own natural sebum production. Even though it's referred to as an oil, it's actually more of a liquid wax (it's extracted from a desert shrub) and is absorbed quickly without feeling greasy or clogging skin.

PUMPKIN SEED OIL

Densely packed with phytonutrients, essential fatty acids, vitamins and minerals that seal in hydration, this oil leaves skin feeling plump, radiant and buttery soft. Its versatility makes it a true star. All skin types, even breakout-prone, can use it generously: it contains zinc, which can soothe irritation and keep skin looking clear and healthy.

RED RASPBERRY
SEED OIL

Consider this your daytime, summertime, anytime oil of choice. Specifically for sun-exposed skin, red raspberry seed oil provides the first layer of UV protection (in addition to wearing a clean mineral SPF) and is an excellent anti-inflammatory due to its high levels of linoleic acid, an essential building block for strengthening the skin's barrier. Find it in Summer's Bounty Beauty Oil on page 98.

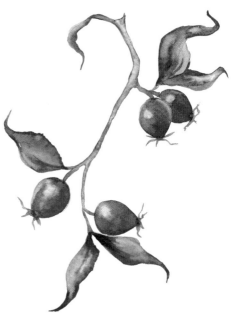

ROSEHIP SEED OIL

This is the oil to turn to when addressing excess melanin hyperpigmentation caused by the sun, hormones or post-acne marks. Omegas, carotenoids, lycopene and vitamin E are just a few of the nutrients you'll absorb from rosehip; the key is to look for oils extracted from both the fruit and the seed. It's also important, as with all plant oils, to source ones that are minimally processed and cold-pressed.

WHITE KAOLIN CLAY POWDER

This detoxifies and draws impurities from the pores while also soothing inflammation and calming hyper-reactive skin. I often use it with clients after a peel or steam. It soothes and nourishes like magic. Keep a white clay mask damp by using a wet washcloth as a facial compress. You never want the clay to fully dry and crack on the skin.

7 FARMERS' MARKET SKIN HEALERS

Sometimes, skincare is as straightforward as a visit to the fruit and veg aisle or a farmers' market. Nature offers what we need to exfoliate, soothe and hydrate skin in these seven simple ingredients:

CUCUMBER

Provides cooling, soothing and healing properties. Its high water content helps to deliver moisture, and reparative vitamin C helps to soothe skin irritations – good to have on hand for minor burns, insect bites and rashes.

AVOCADO

Rich in lipids, antioxidants, minerals and vitamins A, C and E, to hydrate dry and sensitive skin. Avocado can also reduce acne flare-ups, help with wound healing and soothe skin after being in the sun.

PAPAYA

Contains an enzyme called papain, which dissolves and digests dead skin cells. This exfoliation evens skin tone and stimulates your body to produce fresh, plump new skin cells. The papain enzyme can also help with wound healing by keeping bacteria away.

RAW HONEY

The Swiss Army knife of your skincare routine, honey hydrates, tightens, heals and exfoliates the skin. It also helps reduce water loss and has antibacterial properties that protect skin from infection.

STRAWBERRY

High in free-radical-fighting Vitamin C, strawberries are also a natural source of salicylic acid, which helps to decongest clogged pores and works to clear breakouts by preventing dead cell build-up. Try mashing two organic strawberries into a small scoop of raw honey for a quick and easy single-use DIY mask.

TOMATO

Tomatoes are unique because they contain a phytochemical called lycopene, which helps to strengthen your skin's resiliency to UV sun exposure. They're also filled with a potent blend of vitamins and antioxidants that reduce inflammation, repair cellular damage, and soften skin texture. In a high-speed blender, mix half of an organic tomato with a splash of coconut milk until a purée texture is achieved. Massage onto clean skin, enjoy for 15 minutes, and then rinse with cool water.

UNSWEETENED NATURAL YOGURT

Natual yogurt contains naturally occurring lactic acid, which brightens, softens and exfoliates skin.

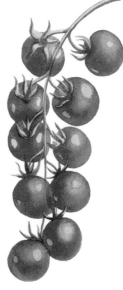

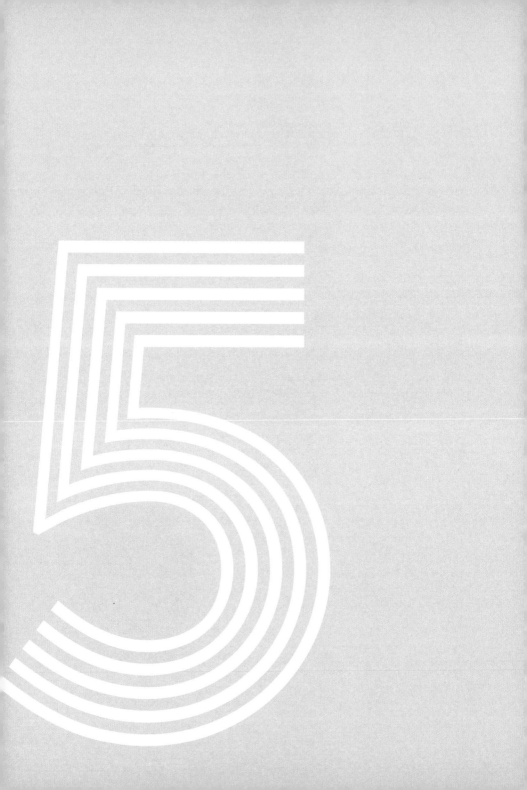

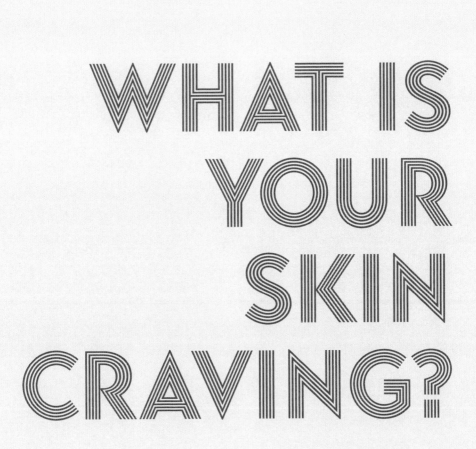

WHAT IS YOUR SKIN CRAVING?

'EACH
MOMENT
OF THE
YEAR HAS
ITS OWN
BEAUTY.'

– RALPH WALDO EMERSON

HOW THE SEASONS AND ENVIRONMENT IMPACT YOUR SKIN

During every season, it's important to listen to Nature and to our bodies to detect subtle shifts. The weather and environment play a major role in overall skin health. Have you ever noticed how your skin feels dewy in more humid climates, and dehydrated in arid ones? These changes in skin seem obvious, but what's not always clear is how to handle environmental conditions that are out of our control. Becoming aware of this seasonal skin connection allows us to nurture and care for our bodies and their often-changing needs. Here are some simple guidelines you can refer to when travelling to new climates and as the seasons change.

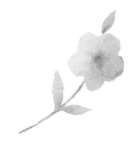

SPRING

We respond to the gentle urges of the sun staying a bit longer in the sky and to the bees that hum as the budding ground is roused to life. We slip again into the beautiful magic that is springtime. **Spring is the season of surrender.** We must tune in and ask ourselves what we need to let go of, in order to feel fully alive and nourished.

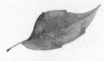

WHEN THE AIR IS POLLUTED

Living in or frequently travelling to environments where the air is polluted causes free-radical damage in the skin. As a general term, you may see this called 'environmental damage' on skincare labels. This refers to any sort of excess oxidation that is caused by exhaust fumes, cigarette smoke, dirt, dust, smog or any other form of air pollution that leaves a residue of impurities on the surface of skin. Sun damage is also a significant type of environmental damage. City-dwellers are often impacted the most by these conditions and can curb the consequences by practising a few preventative measures: always cleanse skin morning and night, and apply topical antioxidants that are high in vitamin C, such as calendula, rosehip, sea buckthorn and blackcurrant oils. Sunscreen is also a must for the UV protection factor, plus it adds another physical protective barrier between the skin and outside pollutants.

SPRING BEAUTY RITUAL

Spring is about surrendering the things that no longer serve us, so what better time to spring clean your make-up bag and skincare stash?

When spring cleaning your beauty products, remember that expiry dates do matter. Read labels and toss anything that has exceeded its expiry date. Products that contain SPF ingredients, such as tinted moisturizers, are especially sensitive. In addition to manufacturers' expiration guidelines, think back to the last time you wore that lipstick shade. Do you absolutely *love* it? If it was more than six months ago, the answer is probably no. Let it go to make room for products that you wear regularly and that make you feel like your best, most beautiful self. Practise doing more with less, finding bliss in simple pleasures, and clearing emotional toxins that may have stagnated through the winter.

SPRING SKIN CRAVINGS

Keep your spring beauty routine simple and uplifting. Your skin is craving floral hydrosols, such as rose, geranium and neroli. These give skin a sip of essential water moisture while also imparting the botanical benefits of the plant petals. Treat your skin to blended water-dense fruits and veggies, such as cucumber and melon – try the Cooling Honey, Melon and Mint Mask on page 138.

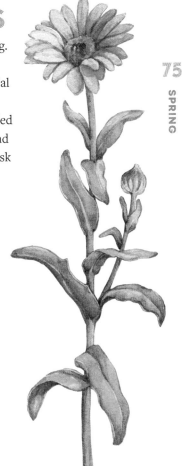

SUMMER

We find joy in dreamy, sunshine-filled days that are long
and leisurely; exposing a bit more of our skin as we seek
the rush of new adventures. We dance to the familiar
soundtrack of crickets at dusk and crashing waves by
the sea. Humidity drapes around our bodies like an unseen
overcoat and we live whole-heartedly in full bloom.
Summer is the season of bounty.

SUMMER BEAUTY RITUAL

If spring is a lesson in minimalism, then summer is the season of excess.
Allow yourself to truly savour and celebrate the fresh decadence of the season
by eating and wearing bright, energetic colours that make you feel beautiful

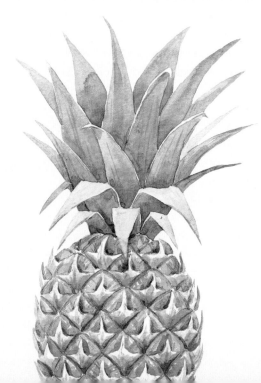

inside and out. Host a simple but meaningful outdoor gathering and have each guest sign up to bring food in a different colour of the rainbow. Someone may bring bright yellow barbecued corn and sliced yellow melon, while another brings purple cabbage coleslaw and juicy red grapes. See how much fun it could be? Aim to wear the colours, too, for a vibrant summer beauty food shindig!

SUMMER SKIN CRAVINGS

Because summer means more sweat and more sunscreen, your skin is craving fresh, seasonal fruits that will exfoliate and renew your skin. Natural fruit enzymes, such as those found in papaya and pineapple, act as mild chemical exfoliants to clear congestion, sweep away sunscreen buildup and keep skin radiant. In addition, aim to use plant oils that contain natural protection from the sun. Some examples include: red raspberry seed oil, carrot seed oil, avocado oil and pomegranate seed oil.

WHEN THE CLIMATE FEELS HOT AND HUMID

This climate is the perfect recipe for congestion and breakouts if excess oil is not balanced. Sweltering conditions cause the skin to feel slick and greasy. While very dry skin types may flourish in this setting, most will enjoy a cooling, clarifying toner such as tea tree, chamomile or lavender, to balance oil and soothe heat inflammation. It is also essential to use a barrier of zinc oxide or titanium dioxide sunscreen to protect skin from the sun.

AUTUMN

Autumn is the season of introspection.
This natural tendency to draw inwards is reflected in our body language: arms hugged tightly around our core, full-tilt forwards, the wind in our hair as we brace fearlessly for chilly air. We begin to crave richer, heavier foods, often ones that evoke childhood memories: some happy, some melancholy. We feel an unspoken urgency for meaning and purpose as we sense another year drawing to an end. Now is the time to pull your energies inwards and focus your attention on gentle self-care.

AUTUMN BEAUTY RITUAL

Like leaves shedding from the trees, now is a great time to buff away excess cellular build-up on your skin with a full body scrub. Draw a warm bath and soak for a few minutes to soften the skin, then use a scrub (such as the London Fog Scrub on page 150 or the Island Healer Manuka Body Polish on page 149), massaging it into skin with gentle circular motions. Start with your feet, ankles and lower legs, then move upwards until you've fully covered your entire body. Be extra tender over your abdomen, and brush in a clockwise direction. You can even scrub your scalp, behind your ears and your lips (which is amazing for the dry, chapped lips associated with this season). If you do choose to scrub your scalp, you may need to shampoo afterwards to remove any oily residue. Leave the scrub on your skin for as long as possible, then sink below the warm water and continue to soak. Stress tension will melt away and your skin will glow with health.

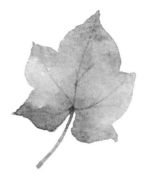

AUTUMN SKIN CRAVINGS

This season is ripe with nostalgic plant-based ingredients to moisturize and protect your skin. Try fresh pumpkin purée smashed with raw honey for an anti-inflammatory exfoliating enzyme treatment, rich in vitamin C. Use pumpkin seed oil to renew skin and help fade and repair summer sun damage. Layer your skincare in the same way you layer your wardrobe for the cooler months. Start with the lightest textures, such as cleanser, hydrosol toner and light plant-based oil, and seal in hydration with a heavier balm. Think of the toner and oil like your trousers and sweater – you wear them everyday; whereas the balm is more to protect your skin from the elements – the outerwear of your skincare 'wardrobe'. These come in especially handy on very windy days or if you know you'll be outside for extended amounts of time, such as when hiking or skiing.

WHEN THE CLIMATE FEELS COOL AND DAMP

This is my favourite weather condition for skin health because skin often retains moisture and has a natural dewy glow. Often, in cooler climates, skin is not exposed to as much sunlight and the risk of UV damage is diminished. In these settings, focus on locking in natural moisture with a few drops of face oil. Refresh skin throughout the day by applying a liberal spritz of hydrating hydrosol toner, such as rose or chamomile.

WINTER

This season is marked by a weary, barren softness.
The trees lift their leafless branches skyward to meet the
cold, twinkling night. We gather with friends and family,
and anticipate the newness that is to come. The fire
crackles in both hearth and heart. We are over-extended
and sometimes exhausted.
Winter is the season of awakening desire.

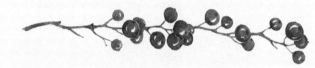

WINTER BEAUTY RITUAL

Buy yourself some fresh flowers to add a bright dose of plant beauty to your space. During this season, we must pay extra attention to stoking our passions, generating warmth and heat in the body (both physically and energetically) and living an intentional beauty-filled life. Seasonal affective disorder can set in as the days are shorter and the weather colder, especially after the thrill of Christmas has ended. Carve out time to write in a journal about what you've accomplished this year and set loving goals for the year to come. If you can write near a window at first light in the morning, this practice will increase clarity and help to balance your circadian rhythm. Don't be afraid to embrace the natural stillness of the season by joining a silent meditation class or by staying in, cocooning yourself in cozy blankets, rather than over-filling your social calendar with Christmas parties. Here are a few journal prompts to get you started:

WHAT AM I TRULY PASSIONATE ABOUT?

WHAT ARE MY VALUES?

WHERE DO I FEEL MOST INSPIRED?

WHAT AM I MOST PROUD OF THIS YEAR?

WHAT SMALL, CONSISTENT ACTIONS CAN I
INCORPORATE INTO MY DAILY ROUTINE TO
HELP ME REACH MY GOALS?

WINTER SKIN CRAVINGS

During this long, dark season your skin craves extra TLC. Look for moisture-binding ingredients that you can whip up to use on your skin, such as avocado, almond milk, cocoa butter and raw honey. Embrace the scents of the season by diffusing essential oils in your home, such as peppermint, cinnamon, clove, grapefruit and ginger. Even though the days are shorter, don't forget your sunscreen. It's a common misconception that you don't need SPF on cold, cloudy winter days, but this extra SPF layer will help to protect you from environmental damage and the cumulative effects of UV exposure.

WHEN THE CLIMATE FEELS COLD AND DRY

If the air outside is dry, you can bet that your skin will soon get sapped of moisture, too. In these cases, the tendency is to over-exfoliate, thinking that dead skin build-up is what's causing your skin to feel rough and dry. In fact, skin needs massage manipulations, warm moist towels, hydrating toner and balm. Gentle exfoliation is important in every climate, so don't leave it out altogether, but do spend extra time massaging skin with an oil cleanser and removing with a warm wet towel. Before the skin has had a chance to dry, liberally mist with a hydrating hydrosol toner and then immediately apply a face oil or balm to seal in the moisture. I also encourage using a humidifier in your room at night, to keep skin soft while you sleep. The same advice goes for arid desert climates that are hot and dry.

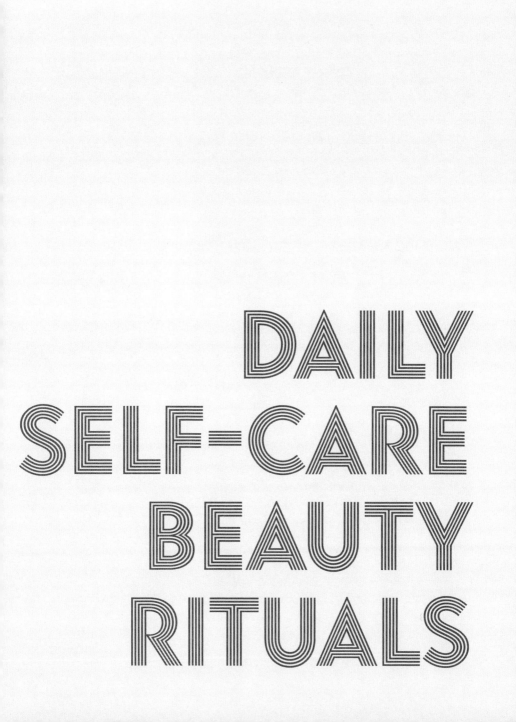

DAILY SELF-CARE BEAUTY RITUALS

MINDFUL SELF-CARE:
A NECESSITY, NOT A LUXURY

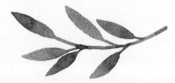

One of my major 'ah-ha' moments came one evening, shortly after I returned home to New York from the work-exchange farm experience. I haphazardly splashed some water on my skin and quickly slapped on a moisturizer. Right then, I realized: *how you do anything is how you do everything.* My careless skincare routine was a direct reflection of how I rushed through everything in my life. Speaking to my husband while looking at my phone screen; hurrying through my morning commute so mindlessly that I didn't even remember making the trip to work; not being fully present on coffee dates with friends.

Take a moment to think about how you truly view self-care. Is it at the bottom of your priority list? Or does it seem too expensive and exclusive? Self-care doesn't have to mean spending hundreds of dollars on spa visits. The truth is: *you hold the power in your own hands* (quite literally) to reduce stress, release negative emotional energy, increase circulation, and revitalize or calm your nervous system. It's time that we reframe the way we think about personal care, understanding that daily habits are a chance to cultivate more mindfulness and inner peace. I've included the following five wellness add-on ideas, which I hope will inspire you to transform your *routine* into a cherished *ritual* that you will look forward to each day.

DRY BRUSHING

Dry brushing, also known as body brushing, is a self-care technique that stimulates the lymphatic system and sweeps away dead skin. It is a sensory experience that energizes your whole body.

The lymphatic system is fascinating. Basically, it is your body's cleanup crew. Through an intricate network of vessels, it collects and transports waste fluid from the tissues to the lymph nodes, where it is filtered before re-entering the bloodstream. It is also responsible for defending you against disease. However, unlike the cardiovascular system, there is no heart-like pump to move the fluid through the body; its movement depends on the natural movements of the body to push it upwards towards its ultimate destination in the veins of the lower neck. That's why regular exercise, massage and manual lymphatic stimulation, such as dry brushing, are important to aid in detoxification. It's also why the direction in which you brush is important.

Follow these simple steps and try devoting 3 minutes each day to this activity for maximum benefits. Dry brushing can be done morning or night, but it feels especially nice in the evening, before soaking in a warm, herbal bath. Dry brushing should feel stimulating, not abrasive, and the bristles should never scratch or break the skin. The best brushes are made from soft natural bristles derived from agave or cactus fibres.

1 Start at your feet and ankles, brushing upwards towards your heart.

2 On your arms, begin brushing at the hands and work upwards, paying attention to the underarm area, where there is a cluster of lymph nodes. Use short upwards strokes, or work in a very gentle circular motion.

3 Brush in a clockwise direction over your stomach.

GUA SHA FACIAL MASSAGE

To continue encouraging lymphatic flow on your face and neck, reach for a Gua sha (pronounced gwa-sah) stone. Gua sha facial massage techniques increase circulation, and engage the parasympathetic nervous system (sometimes called the 'rest and digest' system), which is responsible for slowing heart rate, relaxing muscles and allowing the body time to heal inflammation and digest food.

Gua sha facial massage differs greatly from those used in traditional Gua sha massage bodywork. Using specifically shaped flat polished stones made from jade, rose quartz, nephrite or fluorite, Gua sha brings nutrient-dense blood flow to the skin, unlocks tightly constricted muscles and lengthens fascia, the layer of connective tissue responsible for giving your skin lift and support. It also works to stimulate meridian points, which – according to traditional Chinese medicine – triggers your body's natural healing response, breaks up stagnation or obstructions, and brings balance to the body by allowing energy to flow freely through these internal channels.

I recommend finding a skilled Gua sha practitioner and booking a facial to experience the relaxing, de-puffing magic of this treatment; however, like most things in life, daily Gua sha at home will yield more results cumulatively. After the session, you may ask your skin therapist to give you hands-on instruction for home use. Below are basic guidelines to get you started.

Always perform Gua sha face massage on clean, moisturized skin. Dampen skin with a hydrating toning mist and press 6–8 drops of plant-based oil onto skin, which allows the stone to glide seamlessly over the contours of your face.

The stone should remain nearly parallel (imagine a 15 degree angle) to the skin to capture and sweep fluid just beneath the surface. The stone should never dig into skin or feel uncomfortable.

Perform each step slowly and with intention 3–5 times.

NECK:

1 Sweep the stone up the back of your neck on the right side of the spine, then move to the front of the neck, sweeping the stone from your collarbone to the chin.

CHIN, CHEEK & JAWLINE:

1   Glide the stone from the middle of your chin over your jawline,
    ending the movement at the back of your right earlobe.

2   Place the stone next to the corner of the right side of your lip and
    sweep under the cheekbone, ending at the hairline.

EYES & FOREHEAD

1   Move the stone to the lower inner corner of your right eye and very
    gently sweep under the eye and upwards towards your hairline.

2   Place the stone between your eyebrows and glide upwards to
    the hairline. Then sweep the stone over the hairs of the eyebrow.

3   Repeat steps on the left side, adding a few more drops of oil if
    you ever feel the stone dragging or getting stuck on the skin.

EPSOM SALT BATHS

Hydrotherapy in the form of baths may be the most ancient wellness ritual of
all time. Soaking in a warm bath is one of the most accessible at-home ways
to enhance your routine. Adding Epsom salt (which you can find at your local
chemist or supermarket) to your bath-time ritual soothes sore muscles, helps
to ease monthly menstrual cramps, promotes sound sleep and can lessen the
intensity of common colds. That's because Epsom salt contains magnesium
sulphate, which draws out carbon waste from your pores. Absorbing
magnesium through your bath water is important to overall wellness, as most
people do not get sufficient amounts of magnesium from their diet alone.
Transdermal absorption of Epsom salt is a wonderful way to transform your
bath into a vessel for instant tranquility and long-term health. To elevate your
bath ritual even more, add aromatherapy essential oils and light a few
flickering candles. Recipe ideas for bath soaks can be found in the next
chapter (see pages 146–7).

ACUPRESSURE MASSAGE FOR REFRESHED EYES

Renew tired eyes with this easy-to-learn pressure-point massage, which improves circulation and boosts energy. All of these movements are extremely relaxing and beneficial, especially if you work in front of a computer for long hours or suffer from sinus and tension headaches.

To add an element of aromatherapy, place 1 drop of essential oil on each wrist before performing the pressure-point massage. Lavender, sandalwood, peppermint and sweet orange oils are all excellent choices, or try the Radiant Energy Aromatic Roller (see recipe on page 153), which smells incredible.

Always wash your hands before applying skincare or touching your face for massage.

1   Dispense 2–3 drops of your favourite facial oil and rub vigorously between your palms, both to distribute the product and generate heat in your hands. Use the cushioned pad of your index or middle finger to press firmly on the point above each eye where your eyebrow begins. Press firmly and hold for 3 deep breaths. Repeat 3 times.

2   Next, move to the middle of your eyebrow, repeating the pressure and breathing deeply 3 times; then repeat on the hollows of your temples. You can also use your thumb and index finger to pinch the eyebrow, which releases tension and soothes eyestrain.

3   Drain fluid retention along the lymphatic points under your eyes by gently applying a pulsing pressure directly under the middle of your eye at the very top of your cheekbones. This helps to pump out any fluid that may have stagnated under your eyes and can diminish the appearance of puffiness.

SCALP THERAPY WARM OIL MASSAGE

Champi is an Ayurvedic head massage that is revered in India for the ability to bring vitality and shine to lifeless hair, by increasing circulation to the scalp. Energetically speaking, it helps clear stagnation via the crown chakra at the top of your head to support clear thinking and emotional balance. Massaging your scalp and coating hair strands in warm, plant-based oil feels soothing to your nervous system and is a wonderful way to treat yourself to a beauty ritual that dates back over a thousand years.

The Stress-Free Tresses Warm Oil Ritual recipe (see page 143) utilizes avocado and coconut oils. You can also try using argan, olive or castor oils.

1 Heat the oil in a bowl in the microwave, or in a small saucepan over a low heat, until it reaches a warm and comfortable-to-apply temperature.

2 Using a dropper bottle, dispense the warm oil through the hair, starting at the scalp and massaging through to the ends, until the hair is completely coated. Spend 5 minutes massaging your scalp using the cushioned pads of your fingers.

3 Wrap a hot, damp towel around your head and leave it on for 10 minutes to open the hair shaft and allow the nourishing plant oils to sink deeper.

4 Follow with shampooing and conditioning the hair as usual. You may need to shampoo twice, to ensure that all the oil is thoroughly removed.

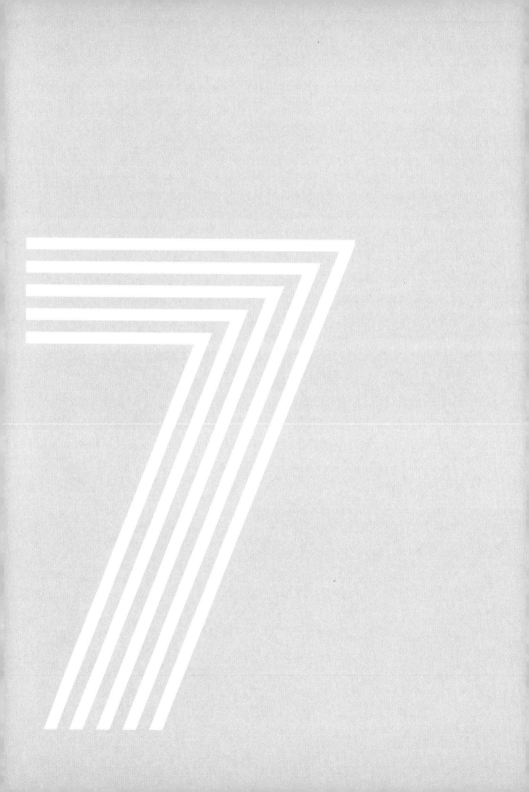

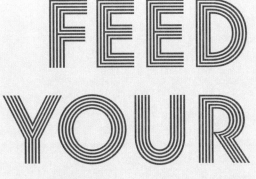

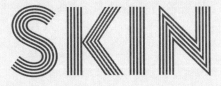

PLANT-BASED BEAUTY RECIPES FOR GLOW GETTERS

In the coming pages you'll discover 50 healthy, non-toxic, plant-based beauty recipes that you can make at home. Some are as basic as blending two ingredients from your storecupboard; some are a little more advanced – requiring warming ingredients in a bain marie (or double boiler), resulting in a longer shelf life.

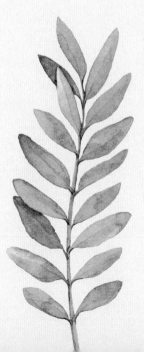

THE ESSENTIALS OF ESSENTIAL OILS

Using essential oils in your skincare routine provides numerous therapeutic benefits, including aromatherapy. They can be utilized in various ways – diffused into the air, added to a warm bath, combined with a carrier oil, applied via facial and body massage, or incorporated into your skincare products.

These plant powerhouses are highly concentrated, quickly evaporating oils, which are generally steam-distilled from the stems, blossoms, leaves, roots, berries, fruits, flowers and bark of various plants. These plant distillations are literally vibrating with life and energy, because they come from living plants that have their own unique energetic properties. Pure essential oils are the direct opposite of lifeless commercial synthetic fragrances that are compounded in a lab.

Essential oils are relatively easy to incorporate into your skincare products as they are lipid soluble, meaning they blend very well with base carrier oils. Each oil has its own unique combination of chemical compounds that lend to a wide multitude of healing benefits.

HOWEVER, WITH GREAT POTENCY COMES GREAT RESPONSIBILITY.

I almost never use essential oils undiluted or 'neat' on the skin and often err on the side of using less than the standard amounts of oils in each product. Often, we think 'if a little bit is good, then more must be better!' This is absolutely not the case with essential oils. Even though they smell divine, a minimalist approach will help you avoid any potential sensitivities or allergic reactions.

CURATE YOUR HOME APOTHECARY

Below is a short reference guide to my favourite essential oils to stock in your home apothecary:

EUCALYPTUS

A refreshing addition to baths; can be diffused in the home to purify the air; natural antiseptic; good addition to healing salves and balms for minor scrapes or insect bites; can be used as a spot treatment for breakouts.

FRANKINCENSE

Precious ancient oil derived from tree resin; great for sensitive, environmentally damaged or acne-prone skin; reduces appearance of stretch marks; can help lessen intensity of raised (keloid) scarring.

GERANIUM

Good for all skin types; equalizes melanin distribution; helps balance hormonal health; a nice addition to face oils and bath soaks.

HELICHRYSUM

A restoring oil excellent for damaged, sensitive skin; regenerative properties; good for fine lines and boosting skin radiance; supports release of emotional stress and tension.

LAVENDER

French lavender is the gold standard; soothes burns, minor cuts and scrapes; good for using on breakouts to cool inflammation and remedy the underlying infection; relaxing aroma with a mild sedative effect; great choice for night-time face oils, bath soaks or room mist to quell restlessness.

PEPPERMINT

Refreshing herbaceous aroma; good for boosting energy levels and uplifting mood; relieves headaches; its cooling sensory effect makes it an ideal addition to carrier oil for a revitalizing foot and leg massage.

ROMAN CHAMOMILE

Soothing, calming effect; beneficial for sensitive, inflamed skin; brings feelings of peace and contentment; helpful when applied topically in facial oils and masks.

ROSE OTTO

A highly valued, expensive oil with a fresh, floral aroma; emollient with skin softening benefits; evens skin tone; nourishing to all skin types; helps relieve feelings of anxiety.

SANDALWOOD

Grounding aroma; good for stimulating the lymphatic system; soothing and moisturizing for dry skin; can be used to cool and lessen the appearance of varicose veins.

THE POWER OF THE PATCH TEST

Never underestimate the power of a patch test. Determine potential reactions on a small, controlled patch of skin (typically the underside of your wrist, behind your ear or the inside crease of your upper arm near the elbow) before you apply the product head-to-toe. Wait 12 hours and if no irritation develops then the product is safe to use. This method can be practised with products you buy as well as the ones you make at home.

PLANT-BASED CARRIER OILS

Here's a list of some of my favourite plant-based carrier oils. Collect them all for your home apothecary, or start small with a few of your favourites:

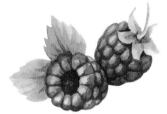

APRICOT KERNEL OIL

ARGAN OIL

AVOCADO OIL

BLACKCURRANT SEED OIL

BORAGE OIL

CALENDULA OIL

CAMELLIA SEED OIL (TEA SEED OIL)

CARROT SEED OIL

COCONUT OIL

EVENING PRIMROSE OIL

GRAPESEED OIL

JOJOBA OIL

MARULA OIL

MEADOWFOAM OIL

POMEGRANATE SEED OIL

PUMPKIN SEED OIL

RED RASPBERRY OIL

ROSEHIP SEED OIL

SAFFLOWER SEED OIL

SEA BUCKTHORN OIL

SUNFLOWER SEED OIL

SWEET ALMOND OIL

TAMANU OIL

VITAMIN E OIL

WATERMELON SEED OIL

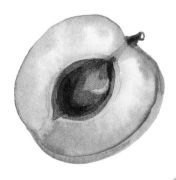

RECIPES
NOT RULES

As much as I'm excited for you to recreate these recipes at home, I'm even more hopeful that you will give yourself creative permission to concoct your own unique new recipes and experiment with ingredients based on accessibility. These raw ingredients are a medium for creating art and inventing new innovative blends that are meaningful and personal to you. The following ideas are guidelines, not hard and fast rules. It's less about 'success' or 'failure' and more about learning and having fun along the way.

PACKAGING AND STORING YOUR PRODUCTS

As you experiment with making your own plant-based beauty products at home, you'll need vessels and a place to store your creations. Storing skincare products in amber or Miron violet glass bottles and jars will help protect them from UV damage from sunlight, thereby extending their shelf life and keeping your ingredients fresh. As a general rule, it's a good idea to store skincare products in a cool place away from direct sunlight, unless refrigeration is required.

RECIPES FOR SENSITIVE SKIN

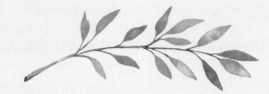

SUMMER'S BOUNTY BEAUTY OIL

With an ingredient lineup this yummy, you'll wonder if it's for your skin or your picnic basket! These fresh fruit and seed oils renew from the outside in and leave skin glowing with health. Use with facial mist (see Rosy Glow Facial Mist on page 120) for best absorption.

MAKES 2 SMALL 30ML (1FL OZ) DROPPER BOTTLES

1½ teaspoons grapeseed oil | 1½ teaspoons watermelon oil

1½ teaspoons red raspberry seed oil | 1½ teaspoons avocado oil

4 drops of rose otto essential oil | 2 drops of neroli essential oil

1 drop of frankincense essential oil

Pour all of the oils directly into a small glass dropper bottle.
Add the essential oils then seal the bottle and swirl gently to mix.

It will keep for up to 12 months in a UV-protected bottle.

To use, press 5 drops into clean, damp skin morning and night.
Use with toning mist for the best results.

ANTI-INFLAMMATORY HEALING BLUE-BLEND BALM

When it comes to soothing skin, this beauty balm is hands-down the best. The essential oil blend is a little more exotic and rare (read: more expensive), but it's so worth the extra cost and effort of sourcing these ingredients. The blue tansy flower is also known as Moroccan tansy. Its oil has antibacterial, anti-inflammatory and skin-calming properties, as well as a show-stopping indigo colour and a sweet, grounding aroma. Helichrysum, also known as Immortelle or Everlasting, is revered as one of the world's most precious healing oils.

MAKES 1 × 60ML (2FL OZ) JAR

1 tablespoon cocoa butter │ 2 tablespoons shea butter
1 teaspoon rosehip seed oil │ 6 drops of blue tansy essential oil
3 drops of helichrysum essential oil │ 3 drops of frankincense essential oil

Scoop the cocoa butter and shea butter into a small heat-safe bowl and set the bowl over a shallow pan of gently simmering water (a bain marie or double boiler) until the butters have completely melted. Remove from the heat and add the rosehip seed oil and essential oils. Stir to blend with a metal spoon, then pour into a wide-necked glass container with an airtight lid. Allow to cool uncovered overnight, then seal with the lid. It will keep for up to 12 months at room temperature.

For dry skin types or chapped skin, apply a pea-sized amount to the face. For acne-prone skin, avoid applying to the face. This balm can also be used on minor burns, scrapes or eczema patches anywhere on the body.

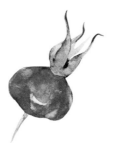

SUN-STEEPED INSTANT CHILL FACE MIST

To make this soothing, toning mist you'll need a preserving (mason) jar and a bit of sunshine! Apply your choice of face oil directly on top to seal in moisture.

MAKES 1 × 200ML (7FL OZ) SPRAY BOTTLE

120ml (4fl oz/½ cup) filtered or mineral water │ 1 × green tea bags
60ml (2fl oz/¼ cup) lavender hydrosol (floral water)

Combine the water and tea bags in a screw-top preserving (mason) jar, seal and leave outside in direct sunlight for 2 hours to infuse.

When the tea has infused, mix it with the lavender hydrosol and pour into a glass spray mist bottle.

Store in the refrigerator for up to 2 weeks and spritz on skin after cleansing or throughout the day whenever your skin needs a refreshing pick-me-up.

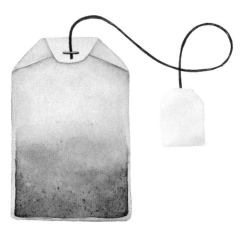

SOFT AS VELVET FACIAL SCRUB

This gentle, granular exfoliant sweeps away cellular build-up and brightens skin thanks to the super-soft rice bran powder. The blend of lavender, rose and blue chamomile works to draw heat and inflammation out of the skin, leaving your face soft and cool to the touch. Your skin will feel refreshed and soft as velvet!

MAKES 1 SMALL JAR

60g (2¼oz/¼ cup) fine rice bran powder (rice bran extract)

3 drops of lavender essential oil | 2 drops of rose essential oil

1 drop of blue chamomile essential oil

2–3 drops of pumpkin seed oil or rosehip seed oil (optional)

Mix the rice bran powder with the essential oils only and stir together until well combined. The mixture should absorb the oil but still remain powdery in look and feel. Place in a glass jar and seal with an airtight lid.

When you're ready to use, scoop a pea-sized amount into your palm, then slowly mix in a few drops of water or toning mist until you have a paste. At this point you could also add 2–3 drops of pumpkin seed oil or rosehip seed oil, if wished. Massage onto damp skin using gentle circular motions. Rinse with cool water and pat dry.

It will keep for up to 12 months at room temperature, if kept sealed and dry.

SIMMER DOWN COOLING FACIAL COMPRESS

There are some days when skin is just angry (think: extra reactive, sunburned, sensitive and irritated). These days call for a calming facial compress to deliver soothing ingredients that will rebalance and reset your moisture barrier. I love this one in particular because oat milk is very skin comforting and the honey acts as a humectant, binding essential moisture to your skin cells.

MAKES 1 COMPRESS

240ml (8fl oz/1 cup) water │ 1 × chamomile tea bag
2 teaspoons raw honey │ 125ml (4fl oz/½ cup) oat milk, chilled

Boil the water, pour over the chamomile tea bag and let steep for 10 minutes. While the tea is still warm, add the raw honey. Let the tea cool overnight or place in the refrigerator.

The next day, add the cold oat milk. Soak a soft cotton or muslin face cloth or chamois (shammy) in the mixture. Wring out excess liquid and apply the cloth to the skin like a sheet mask. Continue re-wetting the cloth and placing on skin for 20 minutes. Afterwards, seal in the moisture with the facial oil of your choice.

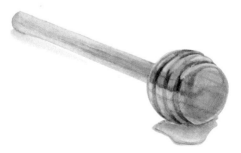

THE SKIN SAVER: WHITE CLAY MASK

Most people think of clay masks as oil-absorbing, moisture-obliterating products for acne-prone skin. Clay does have the ability to draw out impurities, but kaolin white clay is nurturing and gently cleanses without over-drying. This mask is great for all skin types. Use 2–3 times per week.

MAKES 1 ×55G (2OZ) JAR
2 tablespoons white kaolin clay powder
3 tablespoons rose water hydrosol (floral water)
3–5 drops of carrier oil (of your choice)

Mix together the clay powder and rose water hydrosol in a bowl. You can add more clay for a thicker consistency, or more rose water for a thinner paste, to your preference. Stir in the carrier oil. Transfer to a glass container and seal with an airtight lid. Store in the refrigerator for up to a week.

Apply to clean skin with your fingers or (for a truly at-home spa moment) use a mask brush. Let it dry to the point where it feels slightly tacky to the touch (about 10 minutes), then remove with a warm, damp towel.

THE KEY TO DIY CLAY MASKS

Contrary to popular belief, clay masks should NOT be left on the skin to the point where they harden and crack. Even though the sensation of taut skin feels interesting, allowing clay masks to dry out can actually sap skin of moisture and can cause dehydration, even in oily skin types.

The key with clay masks is to keep them slightly moist, which allows the clay to do its work, infusing the skin with valuable minerals. Let clay masks dry to the point where they feel sticky or tacky to the touch, then remove with a warm, damp towel.

ONE-INGREDIENT WONDERS

FRAGRANCE-FREE LIGHTWEIGHT WHIPPED COCONUT FACE CREAM

If your skin is naturally very sensitive or has been environmentally sensitized, it's nice to give your body a break from all kinds of fragrance, including natural essential oils. This is what I call a time of 'fasting' for your skin. If skin is extremely irritated or after having an allergic reaction, consider discontinuing the use of all make-up and skincare for 5 days and instead use only cool water and a tiny amount of this fragrance-free whipped coconut oil cream. Consult a dermatologist who specializes in contact dermatitis and request a patch test if you continue to have reactions once you re-introduce products back into your daily routine.

The most therapeutic coconut oils have been processed very little. The oil should be clear, feel non-greasy and be aroma-free.

MAKES 1 ×225G (8OZ) JAR

200g (7oz/1 cup) cold-pressed organic coconut oil

Place the coconut oil in a mixing bowl. Whip on high speed using a hand-held mixer or vigorously by hand with a wire whisk for 6–7 minutes. The key is to keep the coconut oil cool, so do not heat the oil before whisking. Blend until peaks are formed and a whipped consistency is achieved. Store the cream sealed in an airtight glass container in the refrigerator for up to 12 months.

ALOE VERA MASK

This isn't so much a recipe as it is an encouragement and guide to whipping up your own fresh DIY aloe vera face mask. There's something so satisfying about buying a spiny leaf of aloe vera the length of your forearm, and the assistant at the checkout may well ask you what in the world you intend to do with this natural oddity. Prove your DIY beauty prowess by explaining that you're taking it home to make into a face mask. Prepare for 'oohs' and 'aahs'!

When it comes to raw aloe vera, it's what's inside that counts. The tough spiny leaves encase one of nature's wonders, used for centuries to treat skin ailments. The clear gel-like interior contains active enzymes, amino acids, vitamins and minerals that soothe, hydrate and replenish compromised skin.

MAKES ENOUGH FOR 1 MASK
1 aloe vera leaf

Using a sharp knife, cut the aloe leaf into 8cm (3in) pieces, then make another cut lengthways down the middle of each piece. Open the leaf up and scoop out the clear gel within. Place the gel into a small blender or food processor and pulse until it is completely blended into a frothy jelly consistency.

To use as a mask, apply the mixture to clean face, neck, decollete and upper shoulders. Leave on for 15 minutes, then rinse with warm water. Follow with toning mist and facial oil.

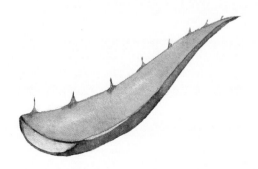

RECIPES FOR BREAKOUT-PRONE SKIN

Soothing breakout-prone skin in the treatment room is one of my favourite parts of being a holistic skincare therapist. It's so incredibly rewarding to hear positive feedback from clients who are slowly seeing acne improvement and feeling more confident in their own skin. Having struggled with painful, ongoing hormonal acne for much of my twenties, I feel a very deep and ever-present empathy for anyone dealing with acne in any form, but especially those with chronic, cystic acne. As I mentioned before, we cannot look at the skin as a standalone entity. All of our systems are related and often the manifestation of acne is one way your body sounds the alarm when something isn't right internally. Looking deeper is almost always the answer; however, making a few lifestyle swaps and using the right skincare are helpful steps on the path to long-term skin health.

ADOPT A NO-PICK POLICY

It's really easy to do more harm than good when you try to extract breakouts on your own. For some, this is a habit that's hard to shake and I often see clients who end up with dark post-inflammatory pigmentation and scarring from picking their skin. If you absolutely must extract a breakout at home, make sure to use a gentle enzyme and warm towel beforehand, to soften and cleanse the skin (the Exfoliating Enzyme Mask Treatment on page 111 is an excellent choice for prepping skin). Also, never use your fingernails. Always wrap your index fingers in clean cotton or use two cotton swabs to gently release pressure and build-up. Remember, your skin's first line of defence is intact, unbroken skin. Be gentle and discerning.

PESKY CULPRITS THAT INTRODUCE BACTERIA TO YOUR SKIN

Observe your own habits. Are you unconsciously touching your face throughout the day without realizing it? Is that mobile phone you have pressed to your cheek regularly cleaned and sanitized? Are your pillowcases and bath towels changed every couple of days? These practices can help to diminish the amount of bacteria on the surface of skin and reduce bacterial breakouts.

IT'S A BREAKOUT, NOT A BLEMISH

Merriam-Webster defines a breakout as 'an eruption or inflammation of the skin'. The definition of a blemish is 'a noticeable imperfection – especially: one that seriously impairs appearance'. See the not-so-subtle difference there? Language is powerful and the words we choose reflect back on us. The term breakout is a matter-of-fact description of what's going on, since acne is an inflammatory condition of the skin; whereas blemish conveys the sense that we are imperfect, defective, deformed or flawed. I never call acne 'blemishes' and I encourage you to be aware of this language, too, both in the way you speak to and about your skin.

SEND LOVE TO YOUR SKIN

It's difficult to feel any gratitude towards your skin when it's inflamed and covered in painful acne. Believe me, I know firsthand. However, ultimately, caring for your skin is more than just applying healthy skincare products topically and feeding your body well. It's also about what you are feeding your mind and spirit. We are so mean to our skin and ourselves. As a result, we often end up mistreating our skin out of frustration and anger. Develop a gentle approach and speak kindly to yourself, especially during the trying times on the path to skin healing. Drink more water. Work up a sweat doing an exercise that you love. Apply your skincare slowly and mindfully. Breathe deeply. Give your skin loving support and time to heal imbalances. Be positive, patient and persistent and know that you are worthy and deserving of radiant, healthy skin.

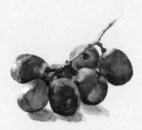

PURIFYING GREEN
CLAY CLEANSER

This clay cream cleanser decongests pores, calms inflammation
from acne, and balances oil production for a healthy, clear glow.
Grapeseed oil is lightweight, aroma-free and non-pore-clogging,
so it makes an excellent choice for acne-prone skin.
Gentle enough for daily use.

MAKES 1 × 55G (2OZ) JAR

3 tablespoons French green clay powder │ 2 tablespoons grapeseed oil
3 drops of tea tree or lavender essential oil (optional)

Mix together the ingredients in a glass jar or pump-action bottle.
You're looking for a viscous, creamy consistency, not a thick paste,
so feel free to add more oil if needed.

Apply with your fingers to skin dampened with warm water,
using gentle circular manipulations. Remove with a wet soft face
cloth (especially if you are removing make-up or sunscreen),
then rinse and pat dry.

SEEKING CLARITY
FACIAL TONER

When it comes to healthy skin, fermentation is your friend. This smelly yet effective toner utilizes fermented apple cider vinegar, which is loaded with natural enzymes and also has antibacterial properties. The addition of lavender essential oil increases the antimicrobial benefits. When skin feels clogged or overly oily, apply this toner with a cotton wool ball after cleansing.

MAKES 1 × 350ML (12FL OZ) BOTTLE

125ml (4fl oz/½ cup) apple cider vinegar | 225ml (8fl oz/1 cup) filtered water

5 drops of lavender essential oil

Mix together the ingredients in a glass bottle, seal and store in a cool place away from direct sunlight for up to 3 months. Does not require refrigeration.

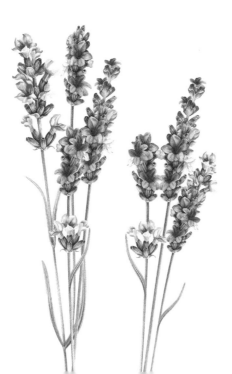

RAPID RECOVERY SPOT TREATMENT

Night-time is when your skin renews, heals and recovers from stress. It only makes sense then to apply an acne-clearing spot treatment overnight, to assist your body's own natural process of healing. Traditional overnight treatments contain harsh, drying ingredients, such as sulphur and benzoyl peroxide, which often irritate already inflamed skin. Gentle white clay paired with tea tree hydrosol helps to heal skin while also destroying the specific bacteria that causes breakouts.

MAKES 1 SMALL JAR
1 teaspoon white kaolin clay powder
½ teaspoon tea tree hydrosol (floral water)

Mix together the ingredients in a small glass jar with an airtight lid. The final product should resemble something of a thick paste, but you may adjust how much tea tree hydrosol you use based on your preferred consistency.

Apply directly to a breakout using a cotton swab. Leave on overnight and rinse clean in the morning.

Keep for up to 1 week in the refrigerator.

EXFOLIATING ENZYME MASK TREATMENT

Papaya contains an enzyme called papain, which works to gently dissolve the sticky protein bonds between dead skin cells, leaving your skin soft and smooth. This natural exfoliation promotes cell turnover, brightens dullness and unclogs congested pores. The addition of finely milled almond flour gives the mask a bit of physical exfoliation property as well, which boosts the results.

MAKES 2 MASKS

70g (2½oz/½ cup) ripe papaya | 1 tablespoon raw honey
½ teaspoon almond flour

In a mixing bowl, mash or blend the papaya into a smooth purée, then add the honey and almond flour. Mix well.

Apply with a gentle circular motion to clean skin, then rinse with warm water.

Use twice a week. You can store any unused mask in the refrigerator for up to 3 days in a sealed glass jar.

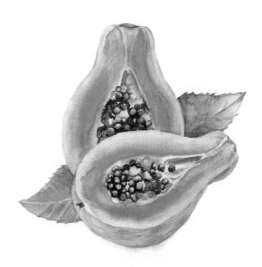

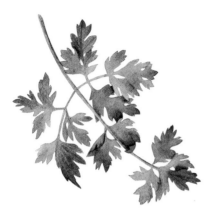

ANCIENT HEALER HERBAL TREATMENT TONER

Before the time of chemists and chic skincare apothecaries, there were skilled herbalists who used plants to treat and heal skin woes. Some of the first written records describing medicinal herbs being used date back to ancient Mesopotamia. Channel your inner Cleopatra by blending these two verdant herbs whenever your skin needs a cooling, anti-inflammatory treatment toner.

MAKES 1 × 225ML (8FL OZ) BOTTLE
225ml (8fl oz/1 cup) witch hazel
6g (¼oz/¼ cup) chopped fresh flat-leaf parsley
6g (¼oz/¼ cup) chopped fresh peppermint leaves

In a small saucepan, heat the witch hazel until almost boiling, then remove from the heat, add the finely chopped herbs, cover with a tea towel and allow to cool completely. Strain through a sieve or cheesecloth and transfer to a glass bottle. Store in the refrigerator for up to 2 weeks.

Apply to clean skin with a cotton pad.

SEEKING BALANCE FACE OIL

Slather your skin in this powerful, breakout-banishing oil to bring balance to your skin and reduce inflammation. Tamanu oil is antibacterial; rosehip seed oil treats uneven skin tone and helps shorten the life of those annoying post-acne red spots that tend to linger long after the breakout is gone.

MAKES 1 SMALL DROPPER BOTTLE

1 teaspoon rosehip seed oil │ ¾ teaspoon red raspberry seed oil
¼ teaspoon tamanu oil │ 3 drops of rosemary essential oil
2 drops of clary sage essential oil │ 1 drop of helichrysum essential oil

Blend together the ingredients and store in a UV-protected glass dropper bottle for up to 12 months.

Press 5 drops into clean, damp skin morning and night.
Use with toning mist for best results.

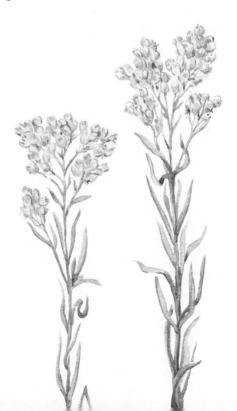

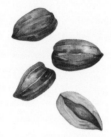

CLEAR GLOW FACE OIL

Jojoba (pronounced ho-ho-ba) is the cornerstone ingredient in this nutrient-dense blend because it's non-greasy and absorbs quickly, even for oily skin types. In fact, it closely mimics your skin's own natural sebum production. That's because technically jojoba seed oil isn't exactly an oil – it's a liquid wax ester, which makes it amazing for balancing oil production without feeling heavy or pore-clogging. Use jojoba with a hydrosol toning mist to lock in maximum moisture. Black cumin seed oil and cypress essential oil help purify, while pumpkin seed oil soothes stressed-out skin.

MAKES 1 SMALL DROPPER BOTTLE

1½ tablespoons jojoba seed oil │ 1½ teaspoons pumpkin seed oil

5 drops of black cumin seed essential oil │ 3 drops of cypress essential oil

10 drops of vitamin E oil

Blend together the ingredients and store in a UV-protected glass dropper bottle for up to 12 months.

Press 5 drops into clean, damp skin morning and night. Use with toning mist for best results.

EXTRA-GREEN GLOW MASK

Whenever you want to channel some serious mermaid vibes, this is the mask for you. Spirulina powder is a next-level antioxidant derived from a blue-green micro-algae, which reverses free-radical damage and also adds a gorgeous deep emerald-green colour to the mask. Bonus point: all of these ingredients are edible and can be added to a yummy smoothie to sip while you wait for the mask to work. You could also add 3 drops of essential oil to the mask; my favourites are mandarin or lemongrass with this particular blend.

MAKES ENOUGH FOR 2 MASKS

1 tablespoon raw honey │ 1½ teaspoons spirulina powder
1½ teaspoons matcha powder

In a mixing bowl, mix the ingredients into a thick, sticky paste.

Apply to clean, damp skin and leave on for 15 minutes. Remove with a warm, soft face cloth (note: the green colour may stain the cloth) or rinse completely with warm water. Follow with toning mist and face oil, to lock in moisture.

Store at room temperature for up to 1 week.

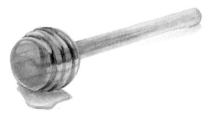

RECIPES FOR HEALTHY, GLOWING SKIN AT EVERY AGE

Ageing should be a celebration, not an ongoing 'battle' that we fear. In many cultures around the world, the elders are revered for their wisdom gained through life experience. However, in the West, it seems ageing has become something we must avoid at all costs... even though it's an inevitable fact of life! In some ways, the external manifestation of ageing skin has become a symbol of our mortality, our brevity and our fragility. And who wants to think about those things? All of this fear around growing older is reinforced by the media and, especially, by beauty brands. Shifting our belief system around ageing and how we talk about it can cause a ripple effect of gratitude. May we acknowledge growing older as a wonderful, beautiful opportunity for a full, vibrant life.

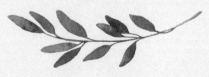

Even with a more conscious mindset, there are biological facts to consider when we address maturing skin. For example, the rate at which your body naturally sheds skin cells slows down; therefore, with more life experience comes the need for more exfoliation to keep skin soft and supple. We must also consider our daily cumulative habits and environmental aggressors that

'TO STAY YOUNG, TO SAVE THE WORLD, BREAK THE MIRROR.'

NANAO SAKAKI

speed up the signs of skin ageing. In our ever-connected digital era, there is a whole new breed of ageing effects caused by high-energy visible blue light from screens. This compounded daily exposure weakens the skin's barrier function and causes oxidative damage. There's also a condition that has been dubbed 'tech neck', which refers to the creasing and fine lines around the chin and neck caused by repeatedly tilting the head downwards to look at screens and devices. In addition to causing unwanted changes in the skin, these patterns disrupt your natural sleep cycle. To get the most benefit from beauty sleep, I recommend powering down at least an hour before bed and aiming not to sleep with the phone in your bedroom.

FACIAL CLEANSING
OIL BASE

When I worked in New York's West Village, I often walked by a little apothecary specializing in exotic essential oils from around the world. Stepping inside was like entering another realm. The woman who worked there was insanely knowledgeable and travelled across continents to source the purest plant oils. Once, I commissioned her to create a customised cleansing oil and was surprised to learn that castor oil is one of the best pre-cleansing oils for removing eye make-up, because of its ability to encourage the growth of healthy brows and lashes. Consider this a cleansing oil base. You can use it as is, without any additions, or you may choose to add in a few drops of lavender, jasmine, rose or your own favourite essential oil blend.

MAKES 1 × 60ML (2FL OZ) BOTTLE

2 tablespoons castor oil │ **1 tablespoon grape seed oil**

1½ teaspoons vitamin E oil

Blend together the ingredients in a UV-protected pump-action glass bottle. Store at room temperature for up to 12 months.

Massage onto dry skin and remove with a warm, damp face cloth.

PETAL PERFECT FLORAL FACIAL STEAM

Facial steaming feels indulgent and leaves a lovely lingering aroma in your home for hours. My favourite way to make this steam is by using dried flowers and herbs, which you can purchase in bulk online, but it can also be made more quickly by substituting the dried material for the essential oil of the same plant. Two drops per plant listed in the recipe should be sufficient. For a gorgeous DIY gift idea, blend the dried herbs and place in a cotton drawstring bag or a clear glass jar.

MAKES ENOUGH FOR 1 STEAM TREATMENT

1 tablespoon dried chamomile flowers │ 1 tablespoon dried rose petals
1 tablespoon dried lavender flowers │ 1 tablespoon dried calendula flowers

Fill a large bowl with 700ml (1¼ pints/3 cups) hot water and add the dried herbs and flowers. Position your face above the steam and place a towel over your head. This helps to soften the skin and delivers the botanical benefits via a relaxing warm steam. Immediately follow with a moisturizing mask or face oil.

You can also steam while wearing an enzyme facial mask – it will activate the enzymes and enhance results.

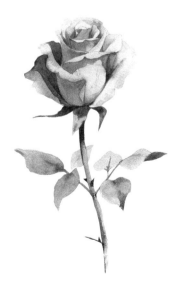

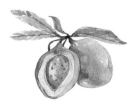

ROSY GLOW FACIAL MIST

Your skin will feel as soft as rose petals after using this ultra-hydrating mist. I absolutely love the aroma of rose, but sometimes in mainstream products it can lean towards smelling too powdery and artificial. Using a purely organic rose hydrosol and high-quality therapeutic-grade essential oil will keep you feeling radiant and smelling rosy.

MAKES 1 × 75ML (2½FL OZ) SPRAY BOTTLE
60ml (2fl oz/¼ cup) rose hydrosol (floral water)
1 teaspoon vegetable glycerine │ 1 teaspoon sweet almond oil
5 drops of rose otto essential oil

Combine the ingredients in a glass spray bottle, shake well, then mist onto clean skin before applying facial oil. Store at room temperature for up to 3 months.

PINEAPPLE ENZYME EXFOLIATING MASK

Nature provides us with powerful exfoliants and one of the most potent exfoliating fruit enzymes for skin renewal is bromelian, derived from pineapple. It decongests clogged pores, refines skin texture and can help brighten hyperpigmentation marks.

MAKES ENOUGH FOR 1 MASK
140g (5oz/1 cup) fresh ripe pineapple (or 2 tablespoons fresh pineapple juice)
1 tablespoon raw honey │ ½ teaspoon almond flour

Using a juicer or a high-speed blender, juice or blend the fresh pineapple. If using a blender, strain the pulp through a sieve or cheesecloth set over a bowl to collect the juice.

Mix 2 tablespoons of the fresh pineapple juice with the raw honey and almond flour and apply to clean skin. Leave on for 10 minutes, then remove with a warm, damp face cloth.

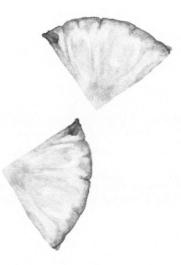

SKIN SOFTENING MICRO=EXFOLIANT

This powder is so fine and soft in texture that it hardly feels like a 'scrub' at all, yet it absolutely does gently whisk away dead skin build-up, without irritating delicate skin. Rice has been used for many centuries across cultures for its brightening, skin-soothing benefits.

MAKES 1 SMALL JAR

2 tablespoons rice flour | 1 tablespoon white kaolin clay powder
1 tablespoon cornflour

Blend together the ingredients and transfer to a sealed glass jar. Store at room temperature for up to 12 months.

To use, scoop a pea-sized amount of powder into your palm and massage onto wet skin. Rinse immediately or leave it on for 5–10 minutes before rinsing. Follow with toning mist and facial oil.

SEEDS OF RENEWAL
FACIAL OIL

This quartet of cold-pressed seed oils delivers vitamins A, C and E and makes skin feel uber-soft and hydrated. It is also filled with flavonoids, antioxidants and essential fatty acids to improve skin elasticity and fight free-radical damage.

MAKES 1 MEDIUM DROPPER BOTTLE

1 tablespoon grapeseed oil | 1½ teaspoons pomegranate seed oil
1½ teaspoons cranberry seed oil | 15 drops of meadowfoam seed oil
10 drops of vitamin E oil

Blend together the ingredients and store in a UV-protected glass dropper bottle for up to 12 months.

Press 5 drops onto clean, damp skin morning and night. Use with a toning mist for best results.

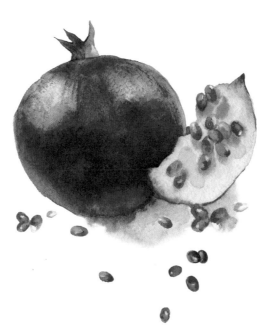

RETIN-ALT NIGHT-TIME REPAIR OIL

If you are looking for a natural, plant-based alternative to traditional retinol, this oil delivers! Carrot seed and sea buckthorn are both packed with beta-carotene, lycopene and a cocktail of skin-protecting antioxidants. Precious marula oil is prized for its ability to mimic your skin's own natural sebum and quickly absorbs into skin without a greasy residue.

MAKES 1 MEDIUM DROPPER BOTTLE

1 tablespoon carrot seed oil | 1½ teaspoons marula oil
1½ teaspoons sea buckthorn oil | 10 drops of vitamin E oil

Blend together the ingredients and store in a UV-protected glass dropper bottle for up to 12 months.

Press 5 drops onto clean, damp skin morning and night.
Use with a toning mist for best results.

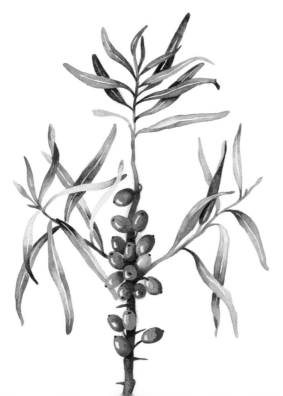

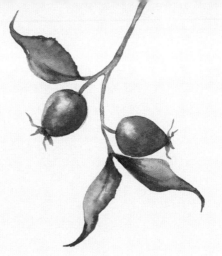

GENTLE EYE SERUM

This blend specifically addresses the delicate eye area, helping to soothe inflammation, detoxify fluid retention and increase circulation to reduce the appearance of dark circles. Infusing the oil in this preparation requires some patience, but the botanical benefits are worth the wait.

MAKES 2 × 100ML (4FL OZ) LARGE DROPPER BOTTLES

125ml (4fl oz/½ cup) jojoba oil | 2 tablespoons organic loose green tea leaves
1 tablespoon dried calendula flowers | 1 teaspoon rosehip seed oil
5 drops of vitamin E oil

Pour the jojoba oil into a glass jar, add the green tea leaves and calendula flowers, then seal with an airtight lid. Let the mixture steep for 4 weeks. This will infuse the oil with the beneficial skin-soothing properties of the green tea and calendula.

When the oil is infused (it may turn a light green colour), strain, then add the rosehip seed and vitamin E oil and transfer to a UV-protected glass dropper bottle.

Apply 2–3 drops under the eyes using gentle tapping motions.
Keep for 12 months in a cool, dry place.

RECIPES FOR MAJOR HYDRATION

MOISTURE BOOST HYDRATING MIST

This refreshing facial toner imparts a gorgeous glow and smells heavenly. Coconut water infused with hydrating glycerine and uplifting geranium is great to use post-gym, after your morning commute or any time your skin needs a boost. Store in the refrigerator during the warmer months and use as a cooling mist.

MAKES 1 × 75ML (2½FL OZ) SPRAY BOTTLE
60ml (2fl oz/¼ cup) coconut water │ 1 teaspoon vegetable glycerine
10 drops of vitamin E oil │ 5 drops of geranium essential oil

Combine the ingredients in a glass spray bottle, shake well, then mist onto clean skin before applying facial oil.
Store in the refrigerator for up to 4 weeks.

CLEANSING CREAM FOR CHAPPED SKIN

Designed to soothe the skin after too much sun exposure or when it feels chapped from winter wind, this cream gently whisks away impurities without stripping the skin's natural protective barrier. If you can't find an accessible calendula hydrosol, substitute with a strongly brewed calendula, chamomile or green tea.

MAKES 1 × 240ML (8½FL OZ) JAR

6 tablespoons sweet almond oil | 6 tablespoons aloe vera juice
1 tablespoon vegetable glycerine | 1½ teaspoons vitamin E oil
3 tablespoons calendula hydrosol (floral water)

Whisk together all the ingredients until well blended and store in a glass container away from sunlight for up to 4 weeks. Shake the jar before each use.

PRO TIP

Freeze any leftover blended aloe vera in ice trays. Frozen aloe feels amazing when applied to minor burns, cuts and scrapes.

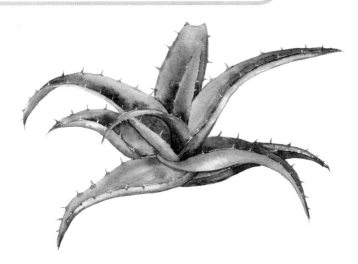

SUPER HYDRATION PROBIOTIC MASK

When you need a cure for dry, chapped skin, reach for this trio of ingredients from your refrigerator. Avocados are rich in vitamins A, D and E, while honey is a humectant that binds moisture to the skin. Look for a full-fat yogurt that contains 'live active cultures', which help to balance the amount of good, protective bacteria in the microbiome on the surface of your skin. Use any leftover ingredients to make a smoothie.

MAKES ENOUGH FOR 1 MASK

½ avocado │ 1 teaspoon honey │ ½ teaspoon natural full-fat yogurt

Blend the ingredients in a bowl until smooth.
Use immediately.

Apply the mixture to the face and neck, leave on for 15 minutes, then rinse with warm water.

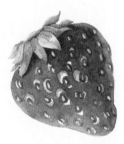

STRAWBERRIES AND CREAM FACE MASK

One of my fondest memories from childhood is visiting the Wimbledon Tennis Tournament with my mother at age 12 and savouring every delicious bite of the iconic strawberries and cream they serve. Who knew that a culinary tennis tradition could also double as a brightening, soothing facial mask? Strawberries are packed with vitamin C and naturally contain salicylic acid to remove dead skin build-up. This recipe is dedicated to you, Mom. And with only two simple ingredients, you can master this one, I promise!

MAKES ENOUGH FOR 1 MASK

3 ripe, organic strawberries | **2 tablespoons natural full-fat yogurt**

In a bowl, smash the strawberries with a fork and mix until as smooth as possible, then mix in the yogurt. Use immediately.

Apply the mixture to the entire face, leave it on for 15 minutes, then rinse with cool water.

THE SWEET TREAT FACE MASK

If your skin had a sweet tooth, this would satisfy every craving. Instead, the mask is beloved by dehydrated skin, as bananas naturally impart vitamin A and potassium to help the skin retain moisture. Cacao powder is high in antioxidants to reverse environmental damage, and almond milk softens rough, dry skin.

MAKES ENOUGH FOR 1 MASK

½ ripe banana | 1 teaspoon cacao powder | 1 teaspoon almond milk

Combine the ingredients in a small blender and blitz. Alternatively, smash the ripe banana in a bowl and whip the other ingredients in by hand. Use immediately.

Apply to the face and neck after cleansing, then rinse with cool water and pat dry.

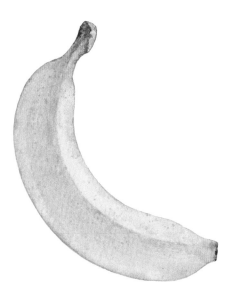

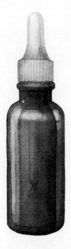

ARGAN AND MARULA FACE OIL

Marula oil is lightweight yet delivers impressive anti-inflammatory, redness-reducing and extremely hydrating benefits. Argan oil has a small molecular size, which allows it to penetrate deeply for maximum moisture payoff. When sourcing, look for cold-pressed oils that have not been processed using high heat.

MAKES 1 SMALL DROPPER BOTTLE
1 tablespoon argan oil | 1 tablespoon marula oil
10 drops of meadowfoam seed oil

Mix together all the ingredients and store in a UV-protected glass dropper bottle for up to 12 months.

Press 5 drops onto clean, damp skin morning and night.
Use with a toning mist for best results.

BLUE DREAMS BEDTIME FACE OIL

Apply this calming blue blend before bed and allow your skin to soak up the benefits while you sleep. Blue tansy adds a deep sapphire hue to the oil and also balances out redness for a more even skin tone. Avocado and grapeseed oil both boost skin elasticity and deliver antioxidants.

MAKES 1 SMALL DROPPER BOTTLE

1 teaspoon avocado oil | 1 teaspoon grapeseed oil
5 drops of blue tansy essential oil | 3 drops of lavender essential oil

Mix together all the ingredients and store in a UV-protected glass dropper bottle for up to 12 months.

Press 5 drops onto clean, damp skin before bed. Use with a toning mist for best results.

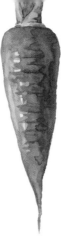

PUMPKIN AND CARROT EXFOLIATING FACE MASK

Pumpkin is a superfood for all types of skin, but especially dry skin, because it contains high levels of zinc, beta-carotene and vitamin C to replenish the nutrients that are depleted through moisture loss. Pumpkin also contains natural enzymes to lightly exfoliate without harsh scrubbing, which dry skin does not tolerate well. You may choose to add the rice bran for an exfoliating boost, or leave it out if your skin is feeling extra dry and irritated.

MAKES ENOUGH FOR 1 MASK

1 tablespoon pumpkin purée | 1 teaspoon organic carrot juice
1 teaspoon raw honey | ½ teaspoon rice bran powder (optional)

In a small bowl, mix together the pumpkin purée and carrot juice, then add the honey and rice bran, if using.

If you want to use it as a warm mask (which feels amazing), place the mixture into a saucepan and warm through over a low heat or place the (microwave-safe) bowl in the microwave for 3 seconds. Apply in gentle circles onto clean skin, then rinse with warm water.

Use twice a week. If not using immediately, store in a sealed glass jar in the refrigerator for up to 3 days.

RECIPES FOR INFLAMMATION

Reactive, inflamed and sensitized skin can manifest from a myriad of causes. Auto-immune disorders, hormone imbalances, digestive inflammation or allergies are just a few of the reasons your skin may be suffering from chronic acne, rosacea, eczema or dermatitis. These conditions can be extremely frustrating and demoralizing. There have been times in my own life when I suffered so much from contact dermatitis and acne that I didn't even want to leave the house. In these cases, it's tempting to try lots of topical products in searching for a solution, when in fact these types of skin issues must be viewed and addressed with a holistic approach. Soothing, anti-inflammatory ingredients will assist your body in healing inflammation; however, they probably are not the end-all answer to these more complex conditions. Seek out a holistic practitioner, naturopath and dietician who can offer a layered strategy and commit to understanding the root cause of your inflammation.

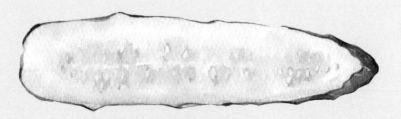

GUIDELINES FOR KEEPING SKIN CALM, COOL AND HAPPY

While you seek out alternative therapies and trace inflammation to the root, here are a few general guidelines to keep your reactive, redness-prone skin happy and calm.

Avoid prolonged sun exposure, as well as any sort of exposure to excess heat. Facial steaming, hot saunas, stimulating or heat-generating skincare products and heat lamps should be avoided at all costs. Skip hot yoga classes and steam rooms at the gym. Heat generated from the sun and these extrinsic sources expands your blood vessels and can cause unnecessary flare-ups in rosacea, histamine reactions and skin irritations.

Synthetic fragrance is *never* your friend, but especially when skin is compromised. Stock your beauty bag with fragrance-free products or natural blends containing very little essential oil.

Don't heat skin from the inside out. Keep heat-generating, pungent foods to a minimum. Some examples include: spicy foods, red wine, tomatoes, peppers, aubergines and citrus fruits. Instead look for fresh, water-dense fruits and veggies such as cucumber, melon, grapes and leafy greens; and soothing spices such as turmeric, fennel and saffron, to cool skin and reduce inflammation.

Focus on repairing and strengthening your skin's natural barrier function by discontinuing the use of alkaline soaps and foaming cleansers that contain surfactants. Don't over-exfoliate skin or use harsh chemical peels. Seek out hydrating ingredients like the ones found in the following six recipes to remedy redness and to calm irritation for balanced, healthy skin.

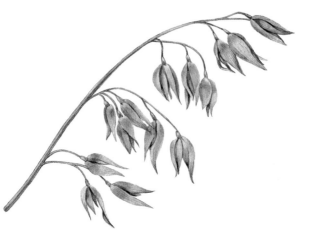

OATMEAL BODY SOAK

Oatmeal is a simple, natural aid for soothing dry, itchy and inflamed skin. I've used this technique to calm my skin during gruelling northeastern winter months and also on my daughter for various skin rashes, eczema and prickly heat.

MAKES ENOUGH FOR 1 BATH
200g (7oz/2 cups) rolled oats

Put the oatmeal into a small drawstring mesh or muslin bag (cheesecloth works, too). Hang the bag under the running tap and draw a warm bath. You can squeeze the bag to more quickly dispense the oatmeal into the water. The water should transform into a silky cloud of skin-soothing goodness. Soak your skin in the bath for 20 minutes and follow with a soothing, fragrance-free body oil.

REISHI MUSHROOM
AND AGAVE MASK

Mushrooms are definitely having a moment. And for good reason!
Reishi mushrooms contain high levels of polysaccharides, which
help skin maintain the water moisture that is essential for renewal
and barrier repair. It's also an antioxidant and anti-inflammatory
ingredient. Agave nectar, derived from succulent desert plants,
helps soothe and soften skin.

MAKES ENOUGH FOR 1 MASK

1 tablespoon reishi mushroom powder │ 1 tablespoon agave nectar
1 teaspoon coconut water

In a small bowl, blend together all the ingredients until smooth.
Use immediately or store in an airtight jar in the refrigerator
for up to 3 days.

Apply to clean skin with fingers or a mask brush. Leave it on
for 15 minutes, then rinse with warm water.

RECIPES FOR INFLAMMATION

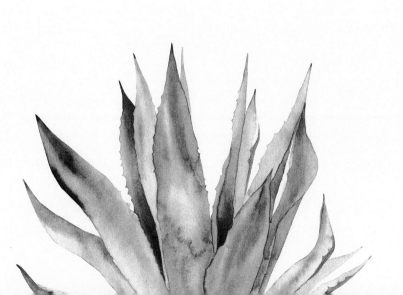

COOLING HONEY, MELON AND MINT MASK

Skin-quenching ripe melon moisturizes and softens skin, leaving it looking dewy and bright. Plus, melon is packed with beta-carotene and vitamin C to repair the skin barrier and encourage cellular turnover. Fresh mint has a herbal cooling effect and is wonderful for taking the heat and sensitivity out of breakouts and insect bites. For an extra-refreshing treat, make this recipe with chilled ingredients so that it goes on cool. Your skin will feel radiant and renewed!

MAKES ENOUGH FOR 2 MASKS

100g (3½oz/½ cup) cantaloupe or honeydew melon, cubed

1 tablespoon coconut milk | 1 teaspoon raw honey

3 fresh mint leaves

Combine all the ingredients in a blender or food processor and blend until smooth. Use immediately.

Apply a thick layer onto clean skin using fingertips or a mask brush. Rinse with cool water and follow with toning mist and facial oil.

Leftovers can be kept in the refrigerator for 24 hours.

BEE'S BOUNTY FACE MASK WITH SEAWEED

Drawing from land and sea, this mask infuses skin with moisture and nutrients from marine minerals to revitalize dry, sensitized skin. Raw royal jelly and honey deliver antioxidants, B vitamins and amino acids to nurture and hydrate for the ultimate skin reset. Avoid using kelp or any kind of seaweed powder if you have marine allergies.

MAKES ENOUGH FOR 1 MASK

1½ teaspoons raw royal jelly | 1 teaspoon raw honey
½ teaspoon kelp powder (or spirulina powder)

Stir the ingredients together in a small bowl until the kelp powder is completely combined. Use immediately or store in an airtight jar at room temperature for up to 2 weeks.

Apply to clean skin with fingers or a mask brush. Leave it on for 15 minutes, then rinse with warm water.

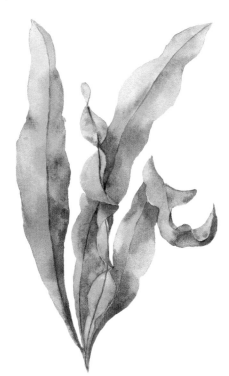

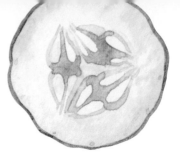

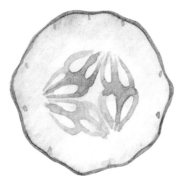

SOOTHING ALOE AND CUCUMBER REFRESHER

Take a quick trip to your local supermarket to pick up the only two ingredients you'll need for this skin-comforting facial mist. The blend of aloe juice and cucumber works wonders for parched, sun-scorched skin. I recommend whipping up a batch anytime you're travelling, but especially for climates that are hot and arid.

MAKES 1 × 250ML (9FL OZ) SPRAY BOTTLE
225ml (8fl oz/1 cup) unsweetened aloe juice, with no additives
½ small cucumber

Combine the aloe juice and cucumber in a blender or food processor and blend until smooth. Strain to remove any pulp or remaining cucumber pieces. Transfer to a glass spray bottle and store in the refrigerator for up to 2 weeks.

SOOTHE AND STRENGTHEN FACE OIL

A minimalist approach to strengthening the skin's barrier function is found in this face oil. Roman chamomile and geranium essential oils help speed up the healing of minor abrasions and diminish inflammation to alleviate itchy, reactive skin.

MAKES 1 SMALL DROPPER BOTTLE

2 tablespoons jojoba oil | 4 drops of Roman chamomile essential oil
1 drop of geranium essential oil

Blend together the ingredients and store in a UV-protected glass dropper bottle for up to 12 months.

Press 5 drops onto clean, damp skin, morning and night. Use with a toning mist for best results.

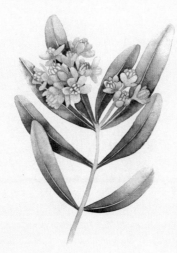

RECIPES FOR HAIR, BATH AND BODY

We place a great deal of focus on the skin of our face, but often neglect everything from the chin down. I always encourage clients not to forget their necks and this advice is true for the décolleté all the way down to your feet. Skin is our largest organ and it's important to exfoliate and moisturize across larger surface areas in order to glow from head to toe. I love the concept of adorning the skin with luxurious aromatic oils. Carving out some time of loving self-care is a powerful energetic act of tenderness to, acceptance of and gratitude for your body – the one that so beautifully carries you through life, just as it is.

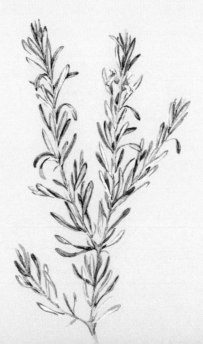

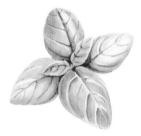

STRESS-FREE TRESSES
WARM OIL RITUAL

This blend is almost too easy, but the silky-soft results are too satisfying not to share! The oil is also deeply moisturizing for the scalp.

MAKES 2 APPLICATIONS (OR 1 FOR ESPECIALLY LONG OR THICK HAIR)
2 tablespoons avocado oil │ 2 tablespoons coconut oil
10 drops of basil, rosemary or clary sage essential oil

Combine the oils in a bowl and apply the blend to clean, dry hair, from root to tip, until completely coated, then comb through.

Wrap the hair in a hot wet towel and leave it on for 30 minutes. The heat helps to penetrate the ingredients and improves hair texture, especially on colour-treated or sun-damaged tresses.

Afterwards, rinse off the oil, then shampoo and condition as usual.

NO-BEACH-REQUIRED TEXTURIZING SEA SPRAY

Your ticket to gorgeous beach hair in a bottle. This easy-to-make hair spritz leaves your locks with lots of volume and a gentle textured wave (and feel free to have fun with the essential oil aromas!).

MAKES 1 × 200ML (7FL OZ) SPRAY BOTTLE

180ml (6fl oz/¾ cup) warm water │ 1 tablespoon sea salt

1 tablespoon Himalayan pink salt │ 1 tablespoon argan, avocado or coconut oil

3 drops of lavender essential oil │ 3 drops of geranium or rose otto essential oil

Pour all the ingredients into a glass spray bottle
and shake to combine.

Spritz liberally onto wet or dry hair. When applying to wet hair,
it's best to let hair dry without the use of heat. Tie hair back or knit
into a loose braid until air dried for effortlessly tousled tresses.

Keep for up to 3 months at room temperature.
Shake well before use.

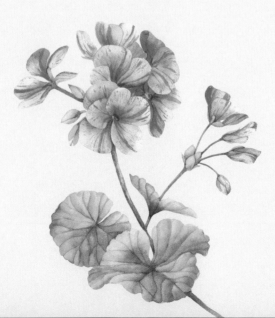

REVITALIZING BROW CONDITIONER

In the same way that the hair and scalp need conditioning, brows and lashes also benefit from moisture. Helping clients to regrow sparse, over-tweezed brows, I often recommend this at-home nightly treatment. Rosemary, lavender and cedarwood all help with rejuvenation and regrowth.

If you leave out the essential oil blend, a small amount of the oil can also be applied to clean lashes. To protect your eyes from potential irritation, NEVER apply essential oils to lashes.

MAKES 1 SMALL DROPPER BOTTLE

2 teaspoons castor oil | ½ teaspoon vitamin E oil
½ teaspoon argan oil | 3 drops of lavender essential oil
1 drop of cedarwood essential oil | 1 drop of rosemary essential oil

Simply combine the oils and pour into your dropper bottle.

Brush into brows using a small lash or brow wand in short upward strokes. The friction from the brush will also stimulate and exfoliate the skin underneath the brows.

Keep for up to 12 months at room temperature.

BATH SOAK: THREE WAYS

Your most luxurious bath, *ever!* These three bath soak recipes help to reduce inflammation and will delight your senses.

For each recipe, simply combine the ingredients and store in a glass jar with an airtight lid. They will keep at room temperature for up to 6 months.

To use, scoop up about 1 cup of the soak mixture and add to a warm bath. Soak yourself in the bath for at least 20–30 minutes for maximum benefit.

MUSCLE MELT BATH SOAK

Arnica is amazing for relaxing overworked muscles and joints after strenuous physical activity – that includes anything from running a marathon or conquering a stressful work week to constantly chasing after a toddler! Sink below the warm water and enjoy 30 minutes of soaking, as muscle tension and stress melt away.

MAKES 1 LARGE JAR (ENOUGH FOR 3 BATHS)

240g (8½oz/1 cup) Epsom salt │ 200g (7oz/1 cup) bicarbonate of soda

200g (7oz/1 cup) sea salt │ 125ml (4fl oz/½ cup) arnica oil

10 drops of rosemary essential oil

SWEET DREAMS
SLEEP SOAK

The magnesium found in Epsom salt promotes sound sleep and can curb feelings of anxiety and restlessness. Paired with sensory calming essential oils, this bath soak will help you sleep soundly and is a supreme act of loving self-care. Pack a small jar when you travel– there's nothing better than checking into a hotel and enjoying a warm, tranquil bath to de-stress you for the fun adventures ahead.

MAKES 1 MEDIUM JAR (ENOUGH FOR 2 BATHS)

240g (8½oz/1 cup) Epsom salt | 200g (7oz/1 cup) bicarbonate of soda
125ml (4fl oz/½ cup) grapeseed oil | 8 drops of mandarin essential oil
5 drops of lavender essential oil | 5 drops of sandalwood essential oil

NO MORE SICK DAYS
BATH SOAK

Body aches and sinus pressure be gone – this soothing soak is designed to get you well *fast*. When you're feeling under the weather, Epsom salt works wonders on the sore muscles associated with cold and flu symptoms. Plus, this therapeutic blend of essential oils will help to decongest nasal passages.

MAKES 1 LARGE JAR (ENOUGH FOR 3 BATHS)

240g (8½oz/1 cup) Epsom salt | 375g (13oz/2 cups) bicarbonate of soda
5 drops of eucalyptus essential oil | 5 drops of vanilla essential oil (or vanilla extract) | 3 drops of tea tree essential oil

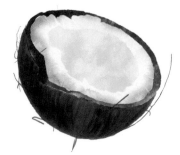

SIMPLE WHIPPED BODY BUTTER

Every DIY beauty enthusiast has at least one body butter concoction in their repertoire. Master this easy recipe and you'll have access to deeply nourishing hydration in minutes. It's also a gorgeous gift idea for mamas-to-be. Make a fragrance-free batch, as here, or get creative and add essential oils to the mix. Use the equal-part volume measurements and you'll be able to commit this recipe to memory forever.

MAKES 1 X 325ML (11OZ) JAR

70g (2½oz/⅓ cup) shea butter │ 90ml (3fl oz/⅓ cup) sweet almond oil
90ml (3fl oz/⅓ cup) coconut oil │ 75g (2¾oz/⅓ cup) cocoa butter

Place the ingredients in a heat-safe bowl and set the bowl over a shallow pan of gently simmering water (a bain marie or double boiler) until the mixture has completely melted. Remove from the heat and set aside until the mixture has partially hardened – you'll see it thicken and become more opaque. (If you are using your own essential oils, this is the point to add them.) Whip the mixture with an electric handheld mixer or with a hand whisk until a fluffy whipped consistency is achieved. Store in an airtight glass jar for up to 12 months.

ISLAND HEALER
MANUKA HONEY
BODY POLISH

This tension-melting restorative scrub exfoliates skin to promote cell turnover, while also healing and hydrating dry, rough skin. The scent is so intoxicating and evokes visions of some far-away exotic island. Manuka honey is a beauty all-star because it draws impurities from the skin while also attracting moisture as a humectant. If Manuka honey is not available, standard raw honey or agave nectar are both great substitutes.

MAKES ENOUGH FOR 5 APPLICATIONS

200g (7oz/1 cup) granulated sugar | 1 tablespoon Manuka honey
1 teaspoon grated fresh root ginger | 60ml (2fl oz/¼ cup) coconut oil
8 drops of ylang ylang essential oil | 4 drops of lemon essential oil

Blend all the ingredients and store in a glass container with an airtight lid for 1 week.

To use, scoop 1 tablespoon of the scrub into your palm, then gently massage onto damp skin during showering or bathing.

LONDON FOG
BODY SCRUB

One of my favourite latte recipes is the 'London Fog', a beautifully scented blend of Earl Grey tea and steamed milk. This recipe is a nod to those delicious ingredients, infusing energizing loose Earl Grey tea with dried milk powder to soften and exfoliate skin. Granulated brown sugar contains naturally occurring glycolic acid, which dissolves dead skin cells for a radiant all-over glow.

MAKES ENOUGH FOR 3 APPLICATIONS

100g (3½oz/½ cup) brown sugar │ 4 tablespoons dried milk powder
60ml (2fl oz/¼ cup) grapeseed oil │ 2 teaspoons Earl Grey loose leaf tea
10 drops of vitamin E oil

Blend all the ingredients and store in a glass container with an airtight lid for up to 6 months. Over time, the oil may separate in the jar; simply stir to mix before each application.

To use, scoop 1 tablespoon of the scrub into your palm, then gently massage onto damp skin during showering or bathing.

FLOWER-INFUSED BODY OIL

There's no doubt that aromatherapy can balance your emotions and mood. When applied, this uplifting botanical blend brings feelings of contentment and gratitude. Perhaps it's the bright yellow calendula flowers steeped in regenerative safflower oil; or the happy scent of sweet orange mixed with jasmine; or maybe it's the rosewood essential oil – a potent aphrodisiac, which uplifts your mood and heightens your senses. Either way, you'll fall in *love* with this body oil.

MAKES 1 × 500ML (17FL OZ) BOTTLE

450ml (16fl oz/2 cups) safflower seed oil

4 teaspoons dried calendula flowers | 8 drops of rosewood essential oil

6 drops of sweet orange essential oil | 4 drops of jasmine essential oil

Pour the safflower seed oil into a glass jar and add the calendula flowers, then seal with an airtight lid. Let the mixture steep for 4–6 weeks.

When the oil is infused, strain then add the essential oil blend and store in a UV-protected glass pump-action bottle.

Apply generously after bathing or showering, while the skin is still damp. Keep for up to 12 months at room temperature.

GLOW=AND=GO
ENERGIZING BODY POLISH

Strong, dark, ground coffee beans add a jolt of stimulating caffeine
to wake up tired senses. It's like a morning cappuccino for your skin!
Cinnamon warms the body for a truly invigorating morning ritual.
Try dry body brushing (see page 85) before applying this scrub
for a double dose of circulation-boosting lymphatic drainage.

MAKES ENOUGH FOR 8 APPLICATIONS

85g (3oz/1 cup) finely ground coffee beans │ 200g (7oz/1 cup) brown sugar
4 tablespoons dried milk powder │ 225ml (8fl oz/1 cup) coconut oil, melted
10 drops of vanilla extract │ ½ teaspoon ground cinnamon

Blend the ingredients and store in a glass container with
an airtight lid for up to 1 month.

To use, scoop 1 tablespoon of the scrub into your palm and gently
massage onto damp skin during showering or bathing.

RADIANT ENERGY AROMATIC ROLLER

Sometimes, you need a midday pick-me-up. Instead of reaching for another cup of caffeine, try this uplifting roll-on aromatherapy blend that will rejuvenate your senses and boost your energy level so that you can power through your day in a mindful, sustainable way.

MAKES 1 LARGE (35ML/1¼FL OZ) OR 3 SMALL (10ML/⅓FL OZ) ROLL-ON BOTTLES

2 tablespoons jojoba oil │ 8 drops of sweet orange essential oil
5 drops of peppermint essential oil │ 3 drops of fir needle essential oil

Blend the oils and store in either 1 large or 3 small glass bottles with rollerball caps.

To use, apply to your pulse points or to the underside of the wrists, behind the ears, at the nape of the neck and on your temples. Avoid the eye area.

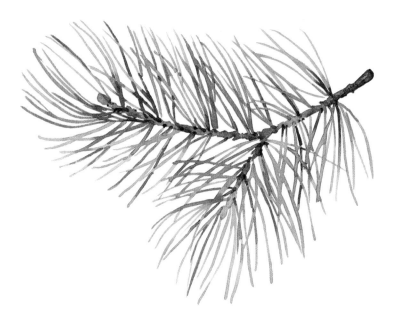

RESOURCES AND FURTHER READING

BOOKS

Absolute Beauty: Radiant Skin and Inner Harmony Through the Ancient Secrets of Ayurveda, Pratima Raichur and Mariam Cohn

Awakening Beauty the Dr. Hauschka Way, Susan West Kurz

The Beauty Chef: Delicious Food for Radiant Skin, Gut Health and Wellbeing, Carla Oates

The Clean Plate: Eat, Reset, Heal, Gwyneth Paltrow

Eat Pretty: Nutrition for Beauty, Inside and Out, Jolene Hart

Renegade Beauty: Reveal and Revive Your Natural Radiance, Nadine Artemis

Sister & Co Skin Food: Natural Skin & Hair Care Treatments, Sophie Thompson

Skin Cleanse: The Simple, All-Natural Program for Clear, Calm, Happy Skin, Adina Grigore

Slow Beauty: Rituals and Recipes to Nourish the Body and Feed the Soul, Shel Pink

Whole Beauty: Daily Rituals and Natural Recipes for Lifelong Beauty and Wellness, Shiva Rose

APPS AND WEBSITES

EWG | Environmental Working Group – www.ewg.org

Think Dirty Shop Clean – www.thinkdirtyapp.com

Good Guide – www.goodguide.com

REFERENCES

ENVIRONMENTAL WORKING GROUP: https://www.ewg.org/
skindeep/2004/06/15/exposures-add-up-survey-results/

ON PARABENS: https://www.ewg.org/skindeep/why-this-matters-cosmetics-
and-your-health/

WASHINGTON POST: https://www.washingtonpost.com/lifestyle/home/
bothered-by-fragrances-this-story-will-be-a-breath-of-fresh-
air/2018/03/19/ace83e8a-26cd-11e8-b79d-f3d931db7f68_story.html?utm_
term=.ac54b1e076dd

ENVIRONMENTAL PROTECTION AGENCY: https://www.epa.gov/indoor-air-
quality-iaq/inside-story-guide-indoor-air-quality

ENVIRONMENTAL HEALTH PERSPECTIVES: https://www.ncbi.nlm.nih.gov/pmc/
articles/PMC2291018/

PICTURE CREDITS

INDEX

ACKNOWLEDGEMENTS

It feels fitting to write a book about beauty when you're blessed with a community of such joy-filled, beautiful people. I couldn't have written this book without the encouragement of my husband Doug Arnaudin. Thank you for taking Anna on so many daddy-daughter dates and allowing me the uninterrupted time to pour hours into this manuscript.

I am extremely grateful for Kate Adams and Sophie Elletson at Octopus Books for their thoughtful editing and intuitive creative direction. Also to the graphic designer, Geoff Fennell, for such a gorgeous cover design and font choices.

To my in-laws Rick and Betsy Arnaudin, and brothers coast-to-coast Ryan and Dave, thank you for always loving me and supporting our family.

Special thanks to my soul-sister Rebecca Casciano for being my most enthusiastic cheerleader throughout this process and for contributing such a lovely foreword. And for their unending confidence and love, Denise Oglesby, Skye Miller, Casey Siljestrom, Brenna Bernabe, Savannah Chase and Kelly Hardee. To Lizzie Anderson, Kimmy Martin and Mary Stoots — better late than never.

Profound gratitude to the Liberty Church family who consistently teach me the power and value in wholeheartedly showing up for your community. Finally, thank you to my mother Rose Knox for being such a lifelong literary inspiration, mentor and friend.